theclinics.com

CLINICS IN PLASTIC SURGERY

Current Trends in Facial Fillers

Guest Editor

DAVID A. JANSEN, MD, FACS

October 2006 • Volume 33 • Number 4

ELSEVIER
SAUNDERS

An imprint of Elsevier, Inc
PHILADELPHIA LONDON TORONTO MONTREAL SYDNEY TOKYO

W.B. SAUNDERS COMPANY
A Division of Elsevier Inc.

1600 John F. Kennedy Blvd., Suite 1800, Philadelphia, PA 19103-2899

http://www.theclinics.com

CLINICS IN PLASTIC SURGERY Volume 33, Number 4
October 2006 ISSN 0094-1298, ISBN 1-4160-4723-9

Editor: Sarah Barth

Clinics in Plastic Surgery (ISSN 0094-1298) is published quarterly by Elsevier Inc., 360 Park Avenue South, New York, NY 10010-1710. Months of issue are January, April, July, and October. Business and Editorial Offices: 1600 John F. Kennedy Blvd., Suite 1800, Philadelphia, PA 19103-2899. Customer Service Office: 6277 Sea Harbor Drive, Orlando, FL 32887-4800. Periodicals postage paid at New York, NY and additional mailing offices. Subscription prices are $291.00 per year for US individuals, $429.00 per year for US institutions, $146.00 per year for US students and residents, $330.00 per year for Canadian individuals, $490.00 per year for Canadian institutions, $353.00 per year for international individuals, $490.00 per year for international institutions, and $174.00 per year for Canadian and foreign students/residents. To receive student/resident rate, orders must be accompanied by name of affiliated institution, date of term, and the *signature* of program/residency coordinator on institution letterhead. Orders will be billed at individual rate until proof of status is received. Foreign air speed delivery is included in all *Clinics* subscription prices. All prices are subject to change without notice. **POSTMASTER:** Send address changes to *Clinics in Plastic Surgery,* Elsevier Periodicals Customer Service, 6277 Sea Harbor Drive, Orlando, FL 32887-4800. **Customer Service: 1-800-654-2452 (US). From outside of the US, call 1-407-345-4000.**

Clinics in Plastic Surgery is covered in *Current Contents, EMBASE/Excerpta Medica, Science Citation Index, Index Medicus, ASCA, and ISI/BIOMED.*

Printed in the United States of America.

CURRENT TRENDS IN FACIAL FILLERS

GUEST EDITOR

DAVID A. JANSEN, MD, FACS
Plastic Surgeon, Private Practice, Metarie, Louisiana; Associate Clinical Professor of Plastic Surgery, Tulane University Medical Center, New Orleans, Louisiana

CONTRIBUTORS

LESLIE BAUMANN, MD, FAAD
University of Miami, Miller School of Medicine, Miami Beach, Florida

TREVOR BORN, MD, FRCS(C)
Plastic Surgeon, Private Practice, Toronto; Associate Staff, Division of Plastic Surgery, University of Toronto, Ontario, Canada

SYDNEY R. COLEMAN, MD
Assistant Clinical Professor, New York University School of Medicine, New York, New York

STEFANIA DE FAZIO, MD
Plastic Surgeon, Private Practice, Naples, Italy

JEFFREY D. FRIEDMAN, MD
Chairman, Institute for Reconstructive Surgery, The Methodist Hospital, Houston, Texas

DAVID J. GOLDBERG, MD, JD
Director, Skin Laser and Surgery Specialists of NY/NJ, New York, New York; Department of Dermatology, Mount Sinai School of Medicine, New York, New York; Fordham Law School, New York, New York

PATRICIO F. JACOVELLA, MD, PhD, FACS
Vice Director, Plastic Surgery Residency and Training Program, Hospital de Clínicas José de San Martín, Buenos Aires, Argentina; Assistant Professor of Plastic Surgery, University of Buenos Aires, Buenos Aires, Argentina

FARAH KHAN, MD
Resident in Plastic Surgery, University of South Florida, Tampa, Florida

GOTTFRIED LEMPERLE, MD, PhD
Clinical Professor, Division of Plastic Surgery, University of California, San Diego, California

PIERRE NICOLAU, MD
Plastic Surgeon, Private Practice, Paris, France

NEAL R. REISMAN, MD, JD
Clinical Professor of Plastic Surgery, Baylor College of Medicine, Houston, Texas; Interim Chief of Plastic Surgery, St. Luke's Episcopal Hospital, Houston, Texas; Attorney at Law, Houston, Texas

RICHARD N. SHERMAN, MD
Skin Institute of New Orleans, New Orleans, Louisiana; Department of Dermatology, Tulane Univesity, New Orleans, Louisiana

CURRENT TRENDS IN FACIAL FILLERS

Volume 33 • Number 4 • October 2006

Contents

FORTHCOMING ISSUES

January 2007

Post-Surgical Breast Reconstruction
Peter C. Neligan, MB, FRCS(I), FRCS(C) and Joan E. Lipa, MD, MSc, FRCS(C), *Guest Editors*

April 2007

Replants and Transplants
Ramazi O. Datiashvili, MD, *Guest Editor*

RECENT ISSUES

July 2006

Gluteal Augmentation
V. Leroy Young, MD, FACS and Thomas L. Roberts III, MD, FACS, *Guest Editors*

April 2006

Abdominal Wall Reconstruction
Mimis Cohen, MD, *Guest Editor*

January 2006

Lipoplasty
Luiz S. Toledo, MD, *Guest Editor*

CLINICS IN PLASTIC SURGERY

Clin Plastic Surg 33 (2006) ix

Preface

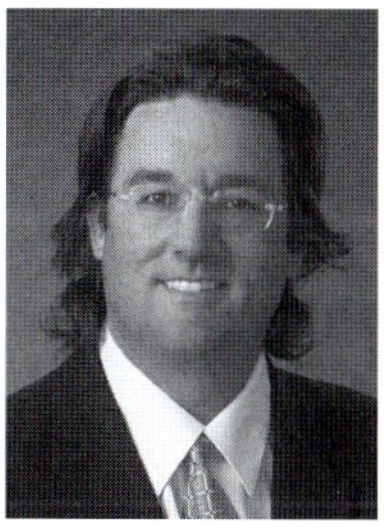

David A. Jansen, MD, FACS
Guest Editor

David A. Jansen, MD, FACS
Private Practice
Metarie, LA, USA

and

Division of Plastic Surgery
Tulane University Medical Center
New Orleans, LA, USA

E-mail address:
djansenmd@hotmail.com

The demand for effective and durable soft tissue fillers has grown dramatically in the last 5 years. As always, plastic surgeons now must compete with many different disciplines for this emerging patient population. This new environment has changed the style, content, and breadth of our plastic surgery practices. We must continuously educate ourselves and our patients on the safe, effective, and durable alternatives in facial rejuvenation.

My own soft tissue journey began in earnest 6 years ago; I began looking for anything that would last longer and perform better than the collagens available. This journey continues with this issue of the *Clinics in Plastic Surgery.*

I have asked the most experienced and published experts across all disciplines to educate both the novice and seasoned injector. Each author was challenged to explain the science behind each filler and give us their precise treatment recommendations and technical pearls for specific areas of the face. Most authors excelled in this request!

There are two articles that delve into the murky medical/legal and ethical waters of facial filler use. Plastic surgeons must combine the scientific, artistic, and ethical elements of each filler to properly educate and treat our patients.

I will be surprised if this issue is not outdated within the next 5 years as the parade of newer and better fillers continues as we go to print. Nevertheless, the principles of filler use outlined in this issue will remain relevant into the future.

It has been an honor to edit this issue of the *Clinics in Plastic Surgery,* and I would like to express my gratitude to Dr. Ruth Owens and Deborah Bordenave for their unending support.

0094-1298/06/$ – see front matter
doi:10.1016/j.cps.2006.10.001
plasticsurgery.theclinics.com

ELSEVIER
SAUNDERS

CLINICS IN PLASTIC SURGERY

Clin Plastic Surg 33 (2006) 505–510

Ethics, Legal Issues, and Consent for Fillers

Neal R. Reisman, MD, JD[a,b,*]

Patient expectations

Patients seek treatments expecting a complete rejuvenation of their facial aging issues. Media and manufacturer marketing help promulgate such views and expectations. Patients would love to have the most minimal treatment that provides them with the most extensive results, and, by the way, NOW. The demand for the magic filler had already been created even before many of the fillers were legally available. Plastic surgeons have a responsibility to establish and accept reasonable expectation standards. We must correct unrealistic expectations; otherwise we may accept liability when we predictably fail to deliver their goal. Conversely, we usually do not want to lose the patient from our care, because the doctor down the street has no problem accepting the patient and guaranteeing these wishful results. This balance between acceptable patient selection and unrealistic patient expectations is the central issue of liability with patients. Patients obtain information from many sources, such as newspaper, television, and other media, usually controlled by the manufacturer. The Food and Drug Administration (FDA) controls what the manufacturer can state, but not what journalists write in their marketing stories. Many exaggerated and false expectations are generated in this fashion. A few of the trendy magazines wrote about Perlane and Restylane before they were granted FDA approval, and Perlane has never received FDA approval. Demand was created in the media before these fillers were available. Patients came to physicians' offices asking for these products, often before the practices were aware of their usage and science. Be cautious about succumbing to patient demand for nonapproved products and patient demands when their goals are unreachable. Fillers can achieve a youthful result, but cannot replace all facial rejuvenation surgery. Patient expectations are difficult to assess unless we specifically ask about their goals. We should honestly describe the filler's longevity and estimate reasonable results. The patient demanding a significant correction of major jowls and severe laxity will not be happy after spending thousands on fillers that do not correct the jowls and extra skin. The patient, despite asking for certain procedures and products, is still the patient, and we as physicians have the responsibility to direct them to reasonable and appropriate alternatives. There are risk managers who believe as long as consents are signed and the patient is informed, choices are permissible. I would suggest

[a] Baylor College of Medicine, Houston, TX, USA
[b] St. Luke's Episcopal Hospital, Houston, TX, USA
* Baylor College of Medicine, 6624 Fannin, Suite 1600, Houston, Texas 77030.
E-mail address: drreisman@hotmail.com

0094-1298/06/$ – see front matter doi:10.1016/j.cps.2006.08.004
plasticsurgery.theclinics.com

that if the expected result is less than stated or desired, liability may attach.

Ethical issues

There may be an ethical dilemma when the patient seeks rejuvenation by fillers and your examination reveals such laxity that only some form of a facelift will correct the deformity adequately. There is an ethical issue in the choice of whether you accept the patient for their desired method or attempt to point out that it will not work and reject their choice, knowing they will be dissatisfied. Some patients will doubt your honesty and believe you are merely attempting to schedule a more costly procedure. They already may have seen your competitor who is willing and happy to do whatever they are asking for regardless of success. The ethical issues arise when a patient seeks a treatment plan the physician knows to be a problem or ineffective. I can make a legal and ethical argument that the physician should know what is best and not perform unnecessary and potentially risky surgery even with a signed informed consent document. Suppose the doctor explains to the pushy patient that their choice of procedure will not correct their concerns adequately. The patient states they want to try it anyway. The legal dilemma now created is that you just explained it will not work, and proceeding makes you appear greedy. If there is a complication, inherent risk, or merely a dissatisfied patient, you may have difficulty in explaining and defending your choices. Once you state an option is not a good choice, it should be a concern then to perform it without additional documentation. Sometimes it is wiser to say no, because you are the person with experience and the patient is seeking an experienced consultation, not merely someone to do what they ask for. Another safe choice, also acceptable, is to document the discussion and proceed with a test area, filling an area of concern. The patient then can evaluate the result and proceed with more, or agree with you and consider more appropriate surgical procedures. One may argue that the successful plastic surgery practice of the twenty-first century must learn mini-surgical procedures to address the large demand for rejuvenation without major surgery and long recovery. Clayton M. Christensen and Michael E. Raynor, in *The innovator's solution: creating and sustaining successful growth* [1], present a historical scenario of modern business failures, (ie, disruption). The established business is disrupted by new companies that possibly address consumer needs and demands better, and not only by offering a lower price. Plastic surgery can be disrupted by failing to adjust to patient demands for lesser procedures with quicker recovery, including fillers and Botox. Not only is it good business to accommodate these demands but also it reduces ethical issues and dilemmas.

Informed consent

Informed consent is a process by which patients learn about their options and choices, the procedure, the product, inherent risks, complications, and required medication-related issues. Once the process is completed, the patient gives consent for what is proposed and documents that they sign a paper. The two national standards are (1) what a reasonable patient needs to know to make an informed decision about his or her care, and (2) what a reasonable doctor needs to tell the patient to make an informed decision about his or her care. Please check with your state as to the required standard and additional requirements. The process of accomplishing this is informed consent, not the signed paper. The signature on the paper merely documents that the patient signed the paper. I believe there should be language indicating the patient understands what the doctor can and cannot do, their questions have been answered, and they elect to proceed (Box 1). I add these exact words into my documented consents or add an additional page the patient acknowledges with a signature. The proposed language is: "I, the patient, understand what Dr. _____ is scheduled to perform, and understand there are no warranties or guarantees. My questions have all been answered and I understanding what Dr._____ can and cannot do, and I elect to proceed."

I believe we can achieve informed consent consistently by using learning styles in our consultations. There are eight learning styles, as defined by Gardner [2]. Three—visual, auditory, and kinesthetic—are the most useful in educating patients. Old studies have stated that only 35% to 50% of what is said to the patient is retained. I believe that this reflects the 35% or so of patients who learn by auditory methods—that is, what is told to them is retained. If we use visual aids and attempt to personalize the consent process, the patient should achieve a much higher understanding of pertinent information. Our consultations should show some schematic or patient pictures that do not establish a warranty, yet honestly depict realistic outcomes, fulfilling visual learner requirements. We should describe accurately and carefully exactly what the filler is, how it works, and what to expect from its use, for those who listen but do not really extract information from pictures. The difficult learning style to address is the kinesthetic learner example. We must try to personalize the description so the patient can understand how they will be affected by the treatment. An example may be to use a Hollywood actor, such

Box 1: **Sample consent (refer to product-specific consents and state law)**

- I authorize and direct ___, MD, with associates or assistants of his or her choice, to perform the following procedure: ___ injection(s) to ___ on ___ for the treatment of ___.
- The details of the procedure have been explained to me in terms I understand.
- Alternative methods and their benefits and disadvantages have been explained to me.
- I understand that the FDA has approved the cosmetic use of ___ for ___. Any other cosmetic use is considered "off-label," but is an accepted and beneficial procedure.
- I understand and accept the most likely risks and complications of ___injection(s) that include but are not limited to: ___.
- I understand and accept the less common complications, including the remote risk for death or serious disability, that exist with this procedure.
- I am aware that smoking during the pre- and postoperative periods could increase chances of complications.
- I have informed the doctor of all my known allergies.
- I have informed the doctor of all medications I am currently taking, including prescriptions, over-the-counter remedies, herbal therapies, and any other.
- I have been advised whether I should take any or all of these medications on the days surrounding the procedure.
- I have been advised that I should avoid aspirin, nonsteroidal anti-inflammatory agents, such as Aleve, Motrin, etc., and wine at least 1 week before my treatment and have complied.
- I am aware and accept that no guarantees about the results of the procedure have been made or implied, and that photos shown are not intended as a guarantee of results or warranty, express or implied.
- I have been informed of what to expect post-treatment, including but not limited to: estimated recovery time, anticipated activity level, and the necessity of additional procedures if I wish to maintain the appearance this procedure provides me.
- If pre- and postoperative photos or videos are taken of the treatment for record purposes, I understand that these photos will be the property of the attending physician.
- I understand that these photos may only be used for scientific or record-keeping purposes.
- The doctor has answered all of my questions regarding this procedure.

I certify that I have read and understand this treatment agreement and that all blanks were filled in before my signature, and I elect to proceed.

________________ ________________

Patient signature/Date Witness signature/Date

_____________ ___________

Print patient name Print witness name

I certify that I have explained the nature, purpose, benefits, risks, complications, and alternatives to the proposed procedure to the patient. I have answered all questions fully, and I believe that the patient fully understands what I have explained.

____

Physician signature/Date

___ copy given to patient ___ original placed in chart

as Melanie Griffith with her "lip addition," or the scene from the movie *First Wife's Club* with Goldie Hawn's new lips. Although not the standard, it gives patients an idea they can adapt to themselves. The more realistic we can make this consultation using these three learning styles, the better the patient's understanding and the more likely we are to have created a loyal patient for the practice. I would encourage the patient to bring photos of what they seek, as well as you discussing excessive fillers using possibly Goldie Hawn in the above movie, Angelina Jolie, or others. Education is strength; rather than selling to patients, educate them about the many available options, the aging process, and which filler may be best, showing your wealth of knowledge in the area. That way you become the expert patients turn to for all information and referrals, rather than seeking whoever can inject the filler du jour. The better the patient's experience in your office, the more loyalty is created for the future.

The team consultation also is appropriate, as long as the doctor is a part of the team. Some states permit nurse practitioners and nurse first assistants to inject fillers without supervision. The actual injector, in those states, has the responsibility to obtain consents. In other states, the physician has the responsibility for at least some of the consent. I believe this is a non-delegable duty that is the physician's responsibility. When a nurse, patient coordinator, or medical assistant does the entire informed consent process, there may be an issue as to the competency of informed consent because the medical assistant is not trained in this and cannot inject the filler alone. It is suggested, therefore, that the practitioner approved to perform filler injections has the duty to accomplish at least a part of the informed consent process. The non-MD performing injections must first comply with state law, in addition to having a specific consent listing that person as the injector. The usual informed consent documentation should be included, but should contain specific reference to the individual actually injecting, avoiding confusion that the MD is performing the procedure when the non-MD is the actual injector.

It is unlikely a malpractice lawsuit claiming lack of informed consent will be successful; a claim usually includes failure to obtain informed consent adding to the negative picture the plaintiff attempts to paint about the physician and practice.

The media reports of Botox parties where patients are seen and then treated, often after champagne, drives risk managers crazy. Similarly, patients who schedule first consultations for fillers should be told to avoid nonsteroidal anti-inflammatory agents, aspirin, wine, and other agents to avoid bruising, as with all procedures. This direction is difficult when the patient is seen for the first time just before treatment. The informed consent process is seldom appropriately completed because the patient usually does not have the time to reflect and ask all questions, or show the consent to friends and family.

Breach of warranty and additional claims

Additional claims, in addition to negligence, often are made in the process of a malpractice lawsuit. The plaintiff's attorney frequently asserts claims not covered by liability malpractice insurance, presumably putting pressure on the defendant to settle the lawsuit. We should be aware of additional claims, such as breach of warranty, breach of privacy, and fraud. Breach of warranty usually is divided into two parts, express warranty and implied warranty. An express warranty may be established when a demonstrable part of the business record is created, such as a photograph, drawing, or similar actual object that represents the stated result to the patient. The practice should be careful in all aspects to avoid such an inclusive representation. Breach of warranty claims do not require that anything be done negligently, only that the promised results were not achieved. This distinction is important because all parties treating the patient performed perfectly, within a standard of care, and nothing negligent occurred. The patient believed a warranty was issued as to a certain result that was not reached. You can see the danger of breach of warranty claims not having the mainstay of medical malpractice, that is, negligence, a part of the claim. In reality, most plaintiffs' attorneys also will claim negligence in some regard to trigger your malpractice insurance defending you and potentially providing settlement or judgment money.

Photographs or demonstrative tangibles made a part of the record that do not include disclaimers may raise this concern. There must be some actual record that claims to establish a warranty as to results. The implied warranty is more of a concern to me. Facts stated during consultation and preoperative visits that the patient and the practice rely on may establish this warranty. Examples are patient statements about a critical meeting, trip, or event that they must attend. If the practitioner hears such a statement, some writing or discussion should take place either to reschedule the treatment or state there is no warranty about results or recovery. Along the same lines, marketing materials should not represent recovery or results that are not obtainable. Patients may seek a specific result using a photo or famous person as a model. Please dispel such ideas, as one cannot and should not guarantee results. All breach of warranty claims have no malpractice coverage and can help lose a defensible lawsuit. A breach of warranty claim is not covered by most medical malpractice insurance, so should one face such a claim, the insurance carrier will most likely issue a reservation of coverage letter stating the company will defend the claim but if there is a judgment or settlement relating to warranty issues the insured will have no protection or coverage. Often plaintiffs' attorneys use this pressure tactic to procure a settlement rather than take the risk for a trial, all part of a malpractice lawsuit strategy.

Privacy issues often are related to disclosure of patient photographs and identity in advertising and office photo books without permission. The Health Insurance Portability and Accountability Act has specific laws governing the authorization of photographs for marketing and these must be followed. Verbal approval and general authorizations usually are inadequate for protection. Specific releases describing the intended use, time, and purpose are suggested.

Fraud issues often are based on withholding information about FDA approvals or critical information necessary for the patient to make an informed decision about care or additional treatment. Misrepresentations and false information on which the patient relies form a basis for these claims. Such false information may include the false FDA status of the chosen filler or misleading information about recovery or complications. The practice should use caution in seeking patients for these treatments and honestly respond to inquiries and estimates on use, longevity, and recovery. All claims and allegations in this section do not have malpractice liability coverage. The surgeon has no insurance coverage and is "bare," placing added pressure for settlement, which fulfills the intent of the plaintiff.

Food and Drug Administration and regulatory issues

The FDA is a regulatory agency for manufacturers but has some interactions with physicians. FDA classifications and our use of drug products are important areas in which we should exercise caution. There are at least three classifications to address. The first is the approved FDA classification. This classification is a good protection for the practice as long as the product is used specifically as the approval states. FDA approval does not eliminate a claim for negligent use and patient treatment, but there is support if there is such approval. Once the product is used in a different area or for a different usage it becomes off-label. This second classification, the off-label usage, generates many opinions today, ranging from complete protection for the physician to absolute illegality. The laws that govern drug-product usage, such as the Federal Food, Drug, and Cosmetic Act [3] and the Controlled Substances Act [4] combine to regulate not only usage but also the interstate transfer of nonapproved products. The physician and practice must understand that off-label protection is not an open approval for usage, but permits physicians to prescribe medications for a different use than that approved by the FDA. Case law dictates, however, that the off-label use not be experimental. That is, usually a peer-approved publication or presentation citing this off-label usage and general acceptance by the medical community should be present. Second, the patient must be informed of the off-label or non-FDA approval status and acknowledge such by documentation. This documentation will not protect the physician in a lawsuit but certainly helps when the court takes judicial notice that the physician has used a nonapproved FDA product that the jury will hear and see. When an off-label usage is being contemplated, therefore, the practitioner should adhere to discussion with the patient and document the patient's acknowledgment, in addition to listing the non-experimental nature of the product's usage. It also is wise to continually review the FDA status of the products we use and those patients ask us to use, because many of them have not received FDA approval for our intended usage. Examples are Sculptra (only approved for HIV patients with atrophy), Radiesse (Radiance) (approved for vocal cord augmentation), and Perlane (not approved). Practitioners should resist the temptation of viewing these off-label fillers and nonapproved fillers as an economic boom. Patients do ask for them, especially when your competitor has no problem suggesting and using nonapproved substances. The nonapproved fillers put practitioners at risk for civil and possibly criminal exposure. State boards of medicine can and do take action when such items are advertised or when there may be a patient or anonymous complaint. The off-label use must be documented with patient acceptance and acknowledgment.

The last hurdle with off-label products concerns the word "prescribe." An argument can be made that when off-label products or drugs are used, the physician must give the patient a prescription for the drug. Off-label physician protections may not apply when the drug or product is administered in distinction to giving the patient a prescription for the drug or product. When physicians actually administer the drug or product, they become distributors and may lose the so called off-label protection. There is a concern that administering off-label or non-FDA–approved drugs or products adds the further liability of being a distributor of contraband, rather than a protected physician dispensing a prescription for an off-label product. Remember which products are approved for what. Botox, FDA approved for glabellar frown lines, is off-label for other areas. Documentation should protect the practice should this be challenged, either in a malpractice arena or by government agencies. A sample consent form would state that the product is off-label and FDA approved for other uses but not FDA approved for this intended use. The use is accepted and not experimental, and after discussions and questions being asked and answered, is recommended and understood by the patient. The patient would document their understanding of this off-label designation. The non-experimental component is best acknowledged by national presentation, journal article, peer-recognized article, or manufacturer representative statement.

The third group of FDA classifications affecting filler usage is the nonapproved status. Drugs and products may be investigated by the FDA in studies for years, yet until approval is achieved their usage is illegal. There is no off-label protection. The use of a nonapproved product exposes the physician and practice to significant fines and possibly criminal prosecution and loss of license. If the patient imports the product from a foreign country where it is approved, and gets through customs, the administering physician still has liability for using contraband. If the physician tries to import such nonapproved products there are significant exposures. First, US Customs can seize the contraband, and even if one is successful in getting it through customs, the transportation of the product to different states violates the interstate commerce and distribution of illegal products that is punishable by civil fine and possibly criminal action. State medical boards can revoke the medical license of those charged and convicted of using illegal substances. Is it worth the risk? Patients seek all alternatives to aging, and as stated the media lists these illegal products as though they were readily available. Caution must be emphasized about succumbing to patient demand. The same patient seeking such usage, if an inherent risk or complication occurs, may file a malpractice suit citing the illegal use of such product. The defense that the patient was told about the FDA status may not help because the physician or practice is the one under product control and the patient is not the knowledgeable party.

Practices should be educated and up to date concerning FDA approval on fillers and other rejuvenation products. The FDA website, http://www.fda.gov, is a help, as are plastic surgery society websites. Patients may read an article about the latest and best filler du jour that may or may not be approved or even available. Manufacturers create the demand before the product approval is achieved. Caution is the most important aspect of safe usage. I do not believe there is an appropriate consent for non-FDA approved products. If the practice or practitioner stated the product was non-FDA–approved, disclosing this to the patient, they knowingly are violating existing law.

Summary

Plastic surgery practices have changed over the years in patient trends and physician patterns. Fillers clearly are sought after and in demand as a rejuvenation tool. The successful practices must adapt to their usage and become familiar with nuances in treatment. Dr. Mark Gorney (personal communication: *Risk Programs*) has said that to avoid malpractice lawsuits, the physician should have no staff, no office, no patients, and no contracts, and maybe then a lawsuit will be averted. Realistically, we require all of the above, so avoidance of liability is adhering to basic principles of sound patient selection, good informed consent, and appropriate choices in treatment, all delivered with a team approach from a proficient and responsible staff.

Further readings

Reisman NR. Legal issues associated with the current and future practice of anti-aging medicine. J Gerontol A Biol Sci Med Sci 2004;59(7):674–81.

Rohrich R, Kinkel J, Reisman N. Use of off-label and non-approved drugs and devices in plastic surgery. Plast Reconstr Surg 2003;112:241–3.

References

[1] Christensen CM, Raynor ME. The innovator's solution: creating and sustaining successful growth. Boston: Harvard Business School Press; 2003.

[2] Gardner H. Frames of mind: the theory of multiple intelligences. 2nd edition. London: Fontana Press; 1993.

[3] Federal Food, Drug, and Cosmetic Act, 21 USC Chapters 3, 5, 9. 1979.

[4] Controlled Substances Act, 21 USC 956(a). 1997.

ELSEVIER
SAUNDERS

CLINICS IN PLASTIC SURGERY

Clin Plastic Surg 33 (2006) 511–523

Calcium Hydroxylapatite Facial Filler (Radiesse™): Indications, Technique, and Results

Patricio F. Jacovella, MD, PhD, FACS*

The concept of beauty has been influenced all over the world and across the history by many factors, including ethnic background, geographic location, and socioeconomic position, among others. Recent trends in clinical aesthetic practice have favored medical techniques that enhance cultural aspects of "attractiveness" and mitigate certain signs of aging, particularly in the face. As time goes by, because of exposure to sunlight, nutritional habits, and genetic patterns in addition to other factors, the skin starts showing the loss of youthfulness, especially in the face.

The most common aesthetic signs of facial aging include visibility of bony landmarks, skin wrinkles, deep furrows, prominence of nasolabial folds, perioral vertical rhytids, ptosis of the oral commissures, and thinning of the lips. These changes arise from the loss of subcutaneous tissue and concomitant thinning of the dermis.

Facial rejuvenation treatments, both surgical and nonsurgical, attempt to improve patients' needs according to their—and likely their communities as well—aesthetic standards.

Many procedures have been described to reverse aging changes and attempt to achieve an acceptable facial rejuvenation. For example, laxity of tissue and redundant skin must be excised. In addition, age-related skin quality features may require laser treatments or chemical peels. To achieve success in aesthetic medical procedures, it is necessary to

Hospital de Clínicas José de San Martín, Plastic Surgery Division, University of Buenos Aires, Argentina
* Av. Cordoba 2351 01120, Buenos Aires, Argentina
E-mail address: pjacovella@elsitio.net

doi:10.1016/j.cps.2006.08.002
plasticsurgery.theclinics.com

have a well-defined concept of beauty and the ability to analyze together the main patient features and his or her desires.

Conventional rejuvenation surgery likely remains the treatment of choice for patients requiring extensive aesthetic facial changes. However, injectable soft tissue fillers are being seen increasingly as an acceptable option in certain specific aging signs, such as glabellar lines, deep nasolabial folds, marionette lines, buccal commissures, perilips wrinkles, and other cases in which the patient needs to enhance some facial features [1,2].

In such cases, fillers appear to provide more "real-time" results, not characterized by extensive swelling and prolonged recuperative periods sometimes found in face lifts and other surgical procedures. Moreover, physicians often find noninvasive facial fillers a nice complement to surgical rejuvenation procedures, such as a face lift, and for nonsurgical procedures, such as laser treatments and chemical peels [1,3].

From an educational viewpoint, the growing demand for minimally invasive procedures suggests the necessity of teaching young plastic surgeons to perform such techniques [4].

For many years, clinicians and investigators worldwide have been looking for the ideal soft-tissue filling material for aesthetic treatment for various areas of the face. The use of such materials began more than 100 years ago, when paraffin was injected [5,6]. Unfortunately, the result was the development of paraffinomas. In 1893, autologous fat transfer was described as another alternative for soft tissue augmentation [6].

Other materials were developed for this purpose, including the synthetic fillers like silicone. Because of many severe complications, injectable silicone has not remained a method of choice [7].

In the early 1970s Stanford University investigators presented a preliminary study on injectable collagen. A decade or so later, in 1984, collagen was approved by the US Food and Drug Administration (FDA) for medical use [8,9]. In some ways, the approval of collagen marked a milestone for aesthetic practice. Its approval also serves as a catalyst for the continuing search for better filler materials for the face.

Classifications of soft tissue fillers

In a comprehensive review of soft tissue filling options, Jansen and Graivier observe that the available products can be classified into different categories: natural filler substances (collagen and hyaluronic acids), autologous fat, fluid fillers (liquid silicone and acrylamides), microspheres from nonresorbable compounds (poly-methyl-metacrilate and human dermal matrix), particulate materials with microspheres of encapsulated hydroxylapatite, and permanent implantable materials (polytetra fluorethylene) [2]. Several investigators have described similar categories as well [1,3,5,6,9,10].

Regardless of the product, the ideal characteristics of soft-tissue filling material have been identified. These include acceptable filler longevity, biocompatibility, nonmigratory possibility, low adverse event profile, and a reasonable cost–benefit ratio [1–3,6,8,11,12].

Synthetic calcium hydroxylapatite (CaHA) is a soft-tissue filler being investigated currently for use in facial aesthetics. This product may offer many of the desirable properties of a facial filler.

Product description

Radiesse™ (Bioform Inc, San Mateo, CA) is a sterile latex-free nonpyrogenic, semisolid, cohesive subdermal, injectable implant, the principal component of which is synthetic CaHA, a biocompatible material that has been in use for more than 20 years in medicine [13,14]. The product is supplied in 1.3-mL and 0.3-mL disposable syringes with Luer-lock fittings [15].

The semisolid nature of the product is created by suspending calcium hydroxylapatite microspheres of 25-μm to 45-μm diameter in a gel carrier that consists primarily of sterile water and glycerin. The gel structure is formed by the addition of a small amount of carboxymethylcellulose (USP). The gel is dissipated in vivo and replaced with soft tissue growth, whereas the CaHA remains at the site of injection [15].

CaHA is biodegradable, following the same metabolic pathway as bone debris resulting from common bone fractures. After 2 to 3 months, the carboxymethylcellulose is resorbed and replaced by collagen. Finally, a gradual breakdown of the particles occurs, until complete phagocytosis is achieved [16–20].

The CaHA microspheres present in Radiesse have the same chemical composition as the inorganic constituent of teeth and bone [13] and exhibit an extensive safety profile. The biocompatibility of CaHA has been tested extensively in preclinical studies and shown to be nontoxic, nonmutagenic, nonantigenic, or irritating [13]. Moreover, clinical, histologic, and electron microscopic findings after in vivo injections have shown excellent tolerance [12].

Biocompatibility studies on CaHA implants all have been characterized by minimal if any, inflammatory response, with no foreign body reaction and without evidence of local or systemic toxicity [13,16]. When injected as small microspheres, CaHA acts as a scaffold that promotes new tissue formation similar to its surrounding environment. Inside soft tissues such as the dermis, deposited particles support fibroblastic ingrowth and new collagen formation, without calcification. In other words, the properties of CaHA mimic the environment into which it is placed. No osseous infiltration has been found [16]. No migration from the sites of injection has been observed. Figs. 1 and 2 show the microspheres and the surrounding tissues.

Regulatory status of Radiesse

Radiesse has already received FDA approval for laryngeal augmentation, soft-tissue marking, and filling/augmentation of dental intraoseous defects and oral/maxillofacial defects. It has been used successfully in urology as a transurethral bulking agent for stress urinary incontinence [21].

Although the use of Radiesse for facial aesthetics in the United States is currently off-label, it does have regulatory clearance for the treatment of vocal cord insufficiency, oral and maxillofacial defects, and radiographic tissue marking [15].

Off-label use of Radiesse has been described in recent publications as well [2,22]. However, the product already has approval for plastic and reconstructive surgery, including soft tissue augmentation for the facial area in the following countries: Argentina, Canada, Israel, Mexico, Romania, Turkey, and all countries within the European Community [15].

Primary indications and conditions of exclusion

Different facial regions can be injected with CaHA to ameliorate or enhance some facial features: glabellar lines, cheeks, tear troughs, nasolabial folds,

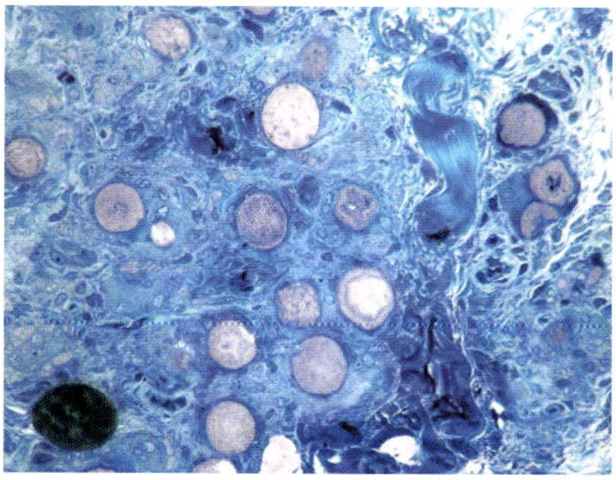

Fig. 1. Optic microscope view: microspherules of CaHA surrounded by thick collagen and histiocytes (arrows). (*From* Marmur ES, Phelps R, Goldberg DJ. Clinical, histologic and electron microscopic findings after injection of a calcium hydroxylapatite filler. J Cosmet Laser Ther 2004;6:223–6; with permission.)

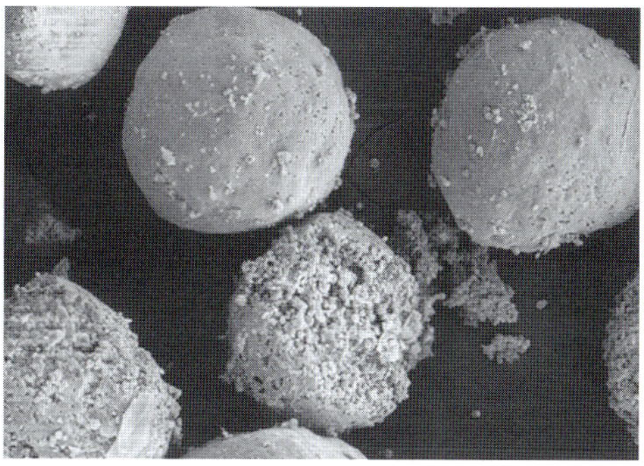

Fig. 2. Electronic microscope view: CaHA particles, 30 months postimplantation. (Courtesy of David J Goldberg, MD, JD, New York, NY.)

nose, lips, marionette lines, oral commissures, chin, and other areas. It is not recommended for crow's feet because crow's feet are in part a consequence of dynamic expression.

In addition, patients with one or more of the following conditions should not receive Radiesse implants: acute or chronic skin infections that involve the site to be treated; existing keloidal scars, systemic collagen diseases, severe bleeding disorders, presence of foreign bodies like silicone, and unrealistic expectations on the part of the patient.

Pretreatment and anesthetic procedures

Preparation

The procedures can be performed in an office setting on an outpatient basis. Patients must provide informed consent for off-label treatment for soft-tissue augmentation before initiation of the procedures. The areas to be treated must be marked appropriately with the patient in an upright position. As with all plastic surgery procedures, pretreatment pictures are mandatory.

Patients must be warned to avoid agents that can produce bleeding, for example, aspirin and some anti-inflammatory drugs, for 7 days before injection. This preventative measure can help minimize hematoma formation [3].

Anesthesia

Depending on the anatomic area, regional infiltrative or nerve block anesthesia (1% lidocaine) may be used. In their didactic report on local and regional block anesthesia, Gmyrek and Dahdah [23] present many interesting guidelines regarding this important subject.

Infiltrative anesthesia has the advantage of a rapid onset of action after injection. Because infiltration of the anesthetic commonly distorts the landmarks of the site, the surgical area to be anesthetized must be identified and marked before injection. In contrast, peripheral nerve blocks are achieved by injecting anesthetic solution around a nerve root to produce anesthesia in the distribution of that nerve.

Nerve blocks are particularly advantageous when infiltration anesthesia may cause unacceptable distortion of the surgical site or require an amount of anesthetic that exceeds the maximum recommended dose. Because most nerves are subdermal, the local anesthetic should be placed in a subcutaneous location. A 30-gauge needle is suggested to deliver the drug. According to the regions to be treated, the following common nerve territories have to be blocked: supraorbital, supratrochlear, infraorbital and mental. Amounts from 1 to 2 mL per zone are enough.

Patient position

Treatments usually are performed with the patient in a sitting or semisitting position, which allows the surgeon to inject the desired sites while effects of gravity affect the skin.

General guidelines for injection of Radiesse

Some factors must be considered when selecting a technique: area to be treated, depth of the injection, and desired injecting volume. The suggested needles are 27-gauge $\frac{1}{4}$ inch long and 25-gauge 1 inch long. The product must be injected subdermally. Intradermal injections can cause visible white nodules in the superficial dermis [16].

Different maneuvers can be used depending on the mentioned factors: linear threading, fanning, and cross hatching. After the needle is introduced in the subcutaneous plane, the product is injected in the created tract during slow withdrawal of the syringe. Needle adaptations may include bending it to access particular contours of the face.

Regarding amounts of Radiesse, as a practical rule it is advisable to gradually achieve the final results over several sessions [3].

Specific injection techniques for specific regions

Glabellar lines

The glabellar wrinkles and furrows develop during the aging process owing to both static and dynamic factors. Such lines typically pose little problem with implants because of the thickness of the dermis and the presence of the underlying connective tissue to support the CaHA.

Even though some hesitation secondary to concerns about tissue necrosis [24,25] and serious complications like embolization [26] have been noted in the literature, no adverse effects have been observed by the author. Nevertheless, caution should be exercised, and treatment of this area by the novice injector is not advised.

A supratrochlear block with 0.5 cc of anesthesia per side is sufficient for this area. To correct the vertical lines, a 27-gauge, half-inch-long needle is used in a linear threading position. The needle is introduced longitudinally in the deep dermis to create a tunnel; the CaHA then is injected into the intradermal-created space by simultaneously slowly withdrawing the syringe and pressing the compound from the syringe into the desired plane. To decrease motion, better results are obtained with a previous treatment with botulinum toxin to weaken the brow depressors [8,16]. The suggested amount of Radiesse is 0.3 mL to 0.5 mL (Fig. 3).

Nasolabial folds

The nasolabial folds are one of the most frequently treated facial areas. The physician should begin by determining the amount of skin redundancy.

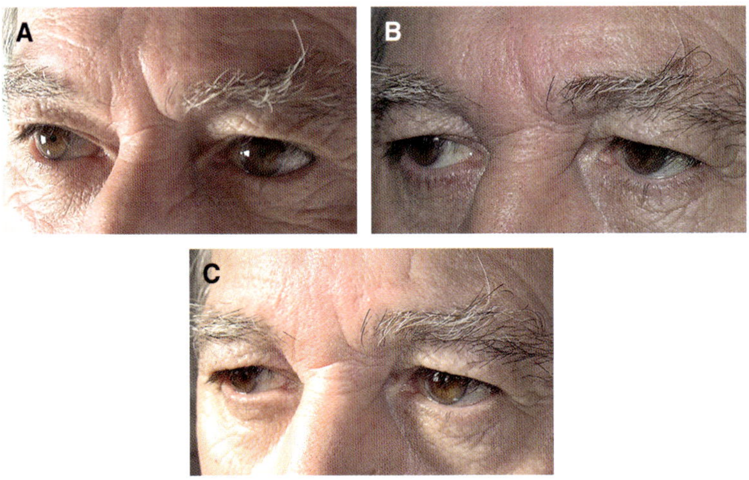

Fig. 3. Pre- (*A*), posttreatment (*B*) at 6-month follow-up, and after 12 months (*C*) in a 64-year-old man with static deep glabellar vertical lines, filled with 0.5 mL in only 1 session.

Depending on the surgeon's experience, if redundancy is too large, a surgical face lift could be considered. Some degree of natural asymmetry is frequent and part of the individual beauty. Special time to observe and identify subtle asymmetries must be taken into account, to be discussed with the patients according to their expectations. After marking the area to be treated, 1 mL of infiltrative anesthesia is injected; a period of 10 minutes postinjection of anesthetic agent before injecting the filler is suggested.

Avoidance of overcorrection is recommended. The product may be injected the first time to achieve a moderate correction and then again with a touch-up 4 weeks later. In the folds, a 25-gauge, 1-inch-long needle is preferred because of the length of the area to be corrected. The needle is introduced along the entire fold longitudinally in a subcutaneous plane. The procedure involves one puncture, starting at the inferior end and terminating near the nose.

Depending on the depth of the folds, 1, 2, or 3 bands of Radiesse must be implanted in parallel rows. There is no need to remove the needle between threads. Suggested volumes are 0.5 mL to 1.5 mL per side [2,8]. The filler material can be massaged and molded to ensure even placement and to avoid an irregular surface appearance. Images in Fig. 4 show the improved appearance in the frontal and three-quarter profile view. The best results are achieved when the abrupt transition from the cheek to the mouth can be effaced [27].

Lips

The lips are considered one of the key features of facial beauty. The ideal lip augmentation procedure should grant predictable results without visible scars. In aging mouth, vertical wrinkles, reduction in vermillion height, vanishing of Cupid's bow, and low lip volume may be considered indications to achieve a better appearance [28]. Therefore, it is important to help the patient define the specific goals of treatment. In addition, the high number of techniques for lip enhancement reflects the lack of an ideal and completely reliable method with predictable and reproducible results. Because of their prevalence in the literature, each of the techniques warrants some mention before any discussion of Radiesse can be considered.

Some complicated surgical techniques, such as dermal flaps [29], may present serious

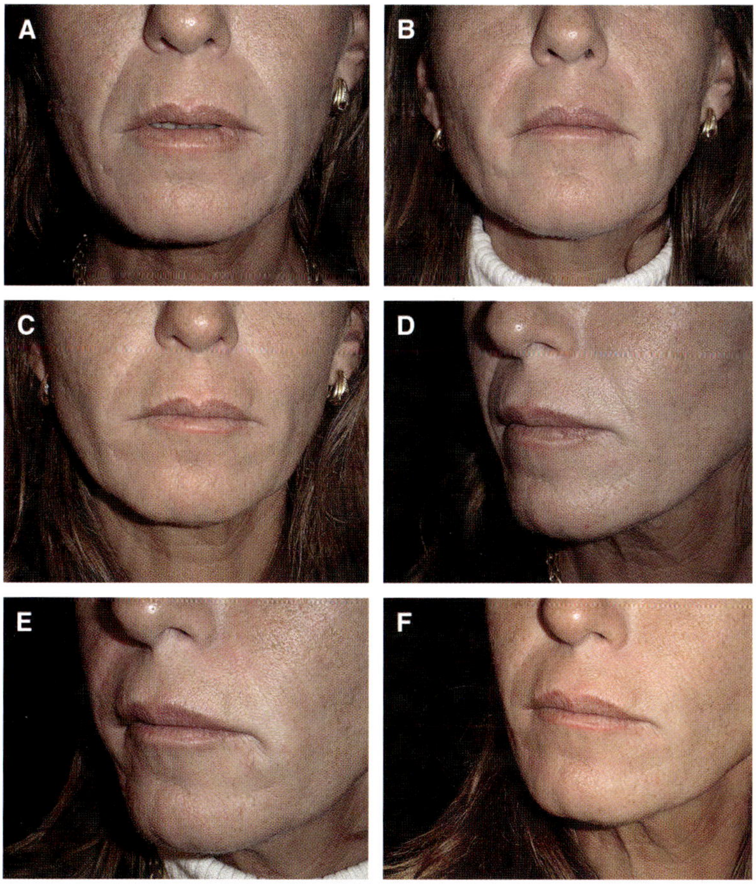

Fig. 4. Deep nasolabial folds (*A, D*) in a 52-year-old woman, treated with 0.5 mL in each side after 12 months (*B, E*) and after 18 months (*C, F*).

complications like asymmetry, noticeable scars, and bridge restriction scars. These scars, if not hypertrophic, can be quite apparent and may necessitate permanent application of camouflage cosmetics.

Leaf and Firouz [30] proposed lip augmentation with superficial musculoaponeurotic system grafts. Most patients expressed some initial concern with their early appearance caused mainly by swelling. Despite corrections remaining for 5 years, the mentioned technique implies 2 surgical procedures, including face lift. It could be considered a good alternative to achieve bulky lips as a complement during major surgery but not for vermillion enhancement.

Polytetrafluoroethylene implants, proposed by Linder [31], offer permanent augmentation results. Sheets of the product can be cut according to necessity in shape and size and introduced thru an incision in the posterior labial mucosa. Despite achieving permanent results, the need for temporary sutures, mandatory 2 days of liquid diet, and possibility of malposition, are considered disadvantages compared with fillers. Dermis fat grafts have been proposed as well and usually provide adequate bulk in the early phase but are unpredictably resorbed over time and may develop fibrotic bands.

Regarding other facial fillers, several compounds can be mentioned. Autologous fat transfer by injection has been proposed for bulking purposes [32]. Such technique has some disadvantages: first, 2 surgical procedures have to be considered, and, second, lasting results are unpredictable, even though some investigators state that it is possible to improve fat permanence by adding endothelial growth factor [33,34]. Because of many complications such as granulomas, serious migration deformities, and systemic reactions, silicone injections should be forbidden [7,35]. Other permanent fillers such as textured silicone particles [36] and polymethylmethacrylate [37] have been used for lip augmentation purposes.

The biggest disadvantage of these compounds is their permanence. If the desired results are not achieved, removal of these permanent fillers is difficult at best and even impossible at times. Because of the greater degree of motion, lip augmentation with fillers is not as forgiving as in the nasolabial region [8]. Therefore, previous training is mandatory. The ideal lip augmentation procedure should grant predictable results without visible scars. Therefore, it is important to help the patient define the specific goals of treatment and analyze probable outcomes before deciding what filler can provide better results [38].

Radiesse can provide long-lasting results up to 18 months without the mentioned drawbacks of both surgical and nonsurgical techniques (Figs. 5 and 6). Treatment of the lips can enhance the lower face and better integrate the perioral area after a face lift [27]. Once again, however, it must be stated clearly that treatment of the lip area should be performed only by surgeons well skilled in their injection techniques in general and with injection of this product in particular.

Nerve block anesthesia is strongly recommended. Infraorbital nerve and mental nerve blocks provide effective anesthesia and reduce the chance of unacceptable distortion sometimes seen in direct infiltration [23]. Proceeding this way, it is possible to achieve a good level of anesthesia with small amounts of lidocaine: 2 mL per side.

A 25-gauge, 1-inch-long needle is selected for this area to limit the number of punctures and to diminish both the incidence of bleeding and hematomas. The preferred plane is between the mucosal border and the orbicular muscle. Two puncture wounds must be created for each side, because each half of the length of the upper lip and lower lip has to be approached from the 2 corners of the mouth. To avoid involuntary spreading, the lip should be held firmly with the thumb, the index finger, and the forefinger while introducing the needle with the other hand. Only 1-layer injections of $\leq$0.5 mL per site are suggested while softly withdrawing the needle. When lip fullness is desired in addition to vermillion enhancement, a deeper second line can be injected. The philtral columns have to be treated separately with a 27-gauge needle.

The total ideal amount is no more than 1 mL for each lip, at least during the first treatment. It is always advisable to begin with low volumes, especially in treatment of the lips [3,27]. To avoid speed bump–like deformities, vertical line fillings should only be performed by experienced surgeons.

Regularly, the linear threading technique itself can help fine radial rhytids to vanish, as the overlying skin stretches out.

Nose

Although conventional aesthetic rhinoplasty remains the treatment of choice for major nasal deformities, injectable facial fillers may provide an attractive alternative in minor defects. Mastery of both nasal anatomy [39] and precise surgical technique [40] is mandatory before performing nasal corrections with fillers. The following anatomic regions can be implanted to improve aesthetic appearance: fronto-nasal angle, dorsum, nasal tip and naso-labial angle.

Patients can be injected once, twice or 3 times, starting always with low volume. As is the case with other areas of treatment with Radiesse, overcorrection is to be avoided. Patients without nasal surgery (Fig. 7) and those who have had previous rhinoplasty (Fig. 8) are suitable for implants. The

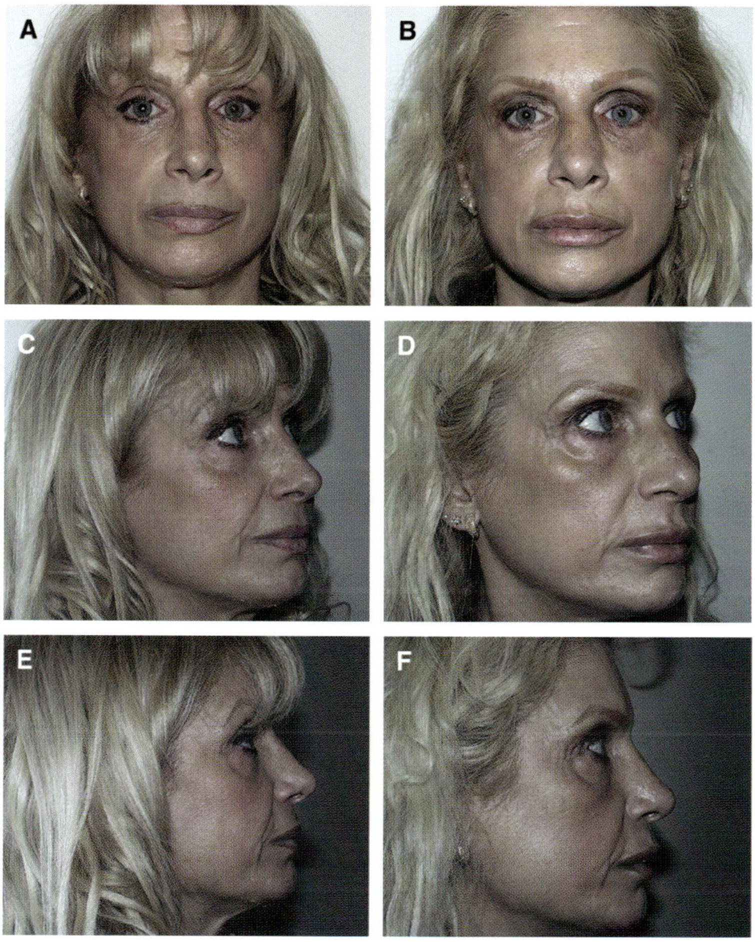

Fig. 5. Pre- (*A, C, E*) and posttreatment (*B, D, F*) of lip augmentation and cheek subtle definition in a 56-year-old woman, treated with 0.8 mL in the superior lip and 0.5 mL in the inferior lip. Postoperative pictures show an enhanced vermilion border and filtrum along with fewer radial lip lines at 12 months. Cheek was treated with 1 mL on each side.

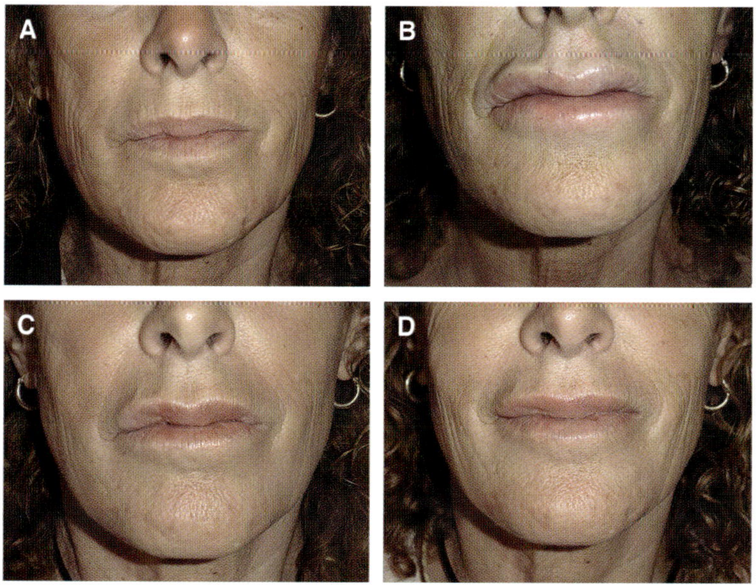

Fig. 6. Pre- (*A*), 24 hours posttreatment (*B*), 12 months posttreatment (*C*), and 18 months' follow-up (*D*) in a 50-year-old woman treated with 0.5 mL in each lip .

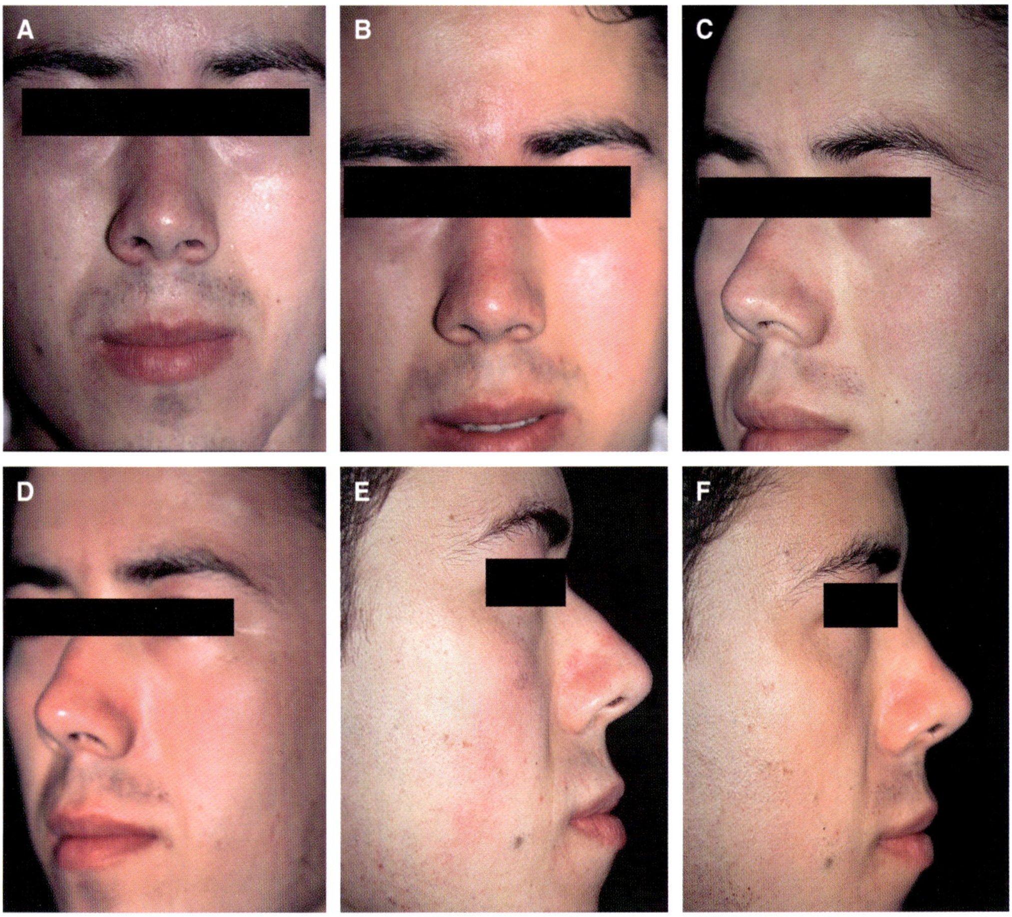

Fig. 7. Pre- (*A, C, E*) and posttreatment (*B, D, F*) of a 25-year-old man without previous surgery of the nose. After 1 mL of Radiesse, the fronto-nasal angle was improved significantly, and conventional surgery was not needed.

suggested maximum volumes for each of the nasal regions are as follows: fronto-nasal angle, 1.5 mL; dorsum, 0.5 mL; tip, 0.5 mL; and nasolabial angle, 1.5 mL.

To avoid distortions, supratrochlear and infraorbital nerve block anesthesia should be applied, and the surgeon should wait 10 minutes before injecting the Radiesse. Proceeding with back and forth multidirectional, using delicate and limited fanning soft movements with a 27- or 25-gauge needle connected to the syringe, the physician can create a subcutaneous space to hold the filler. The product is injected in the previously created space during slow withdrawal of the needle.

The puncture site should be placed distal to the regions to be corrected. Because of the many sebaceous glands in the tip, this area should be approached from the dorsum with a 25-gauge, 1-inch long needle. Microporelike tapes can be applied around the corrected areas to provide desired shape and diminish swelling deformities.

It is very important to clear up that closed and open classical rhinoplasty, with and without autologous cartilage, and Alloderm grafts [41] are still the first option in most nasal deformities. Facial fillers are intended to be an alternative when fast and simple office-based small corrections with the least down time are desired.

Cheek and infraorbital region

Small cheeks and lack of infraorbital projection as individual racial features are very frequent indications for fillers in patients seeking a more youthful appearance. Infiltrative anesthesia can be injected in such areas. A 25-gauge, 1-inch-long needle should be used to approach this area. The puncture site must be distal to the injected region; a cross-hatching technique is preferred to allow adequate spread of the product. The suggested volumes for this area are from 2 to 4 mL, even though 1 mL per side can provide a subtle result (Fig. 5).

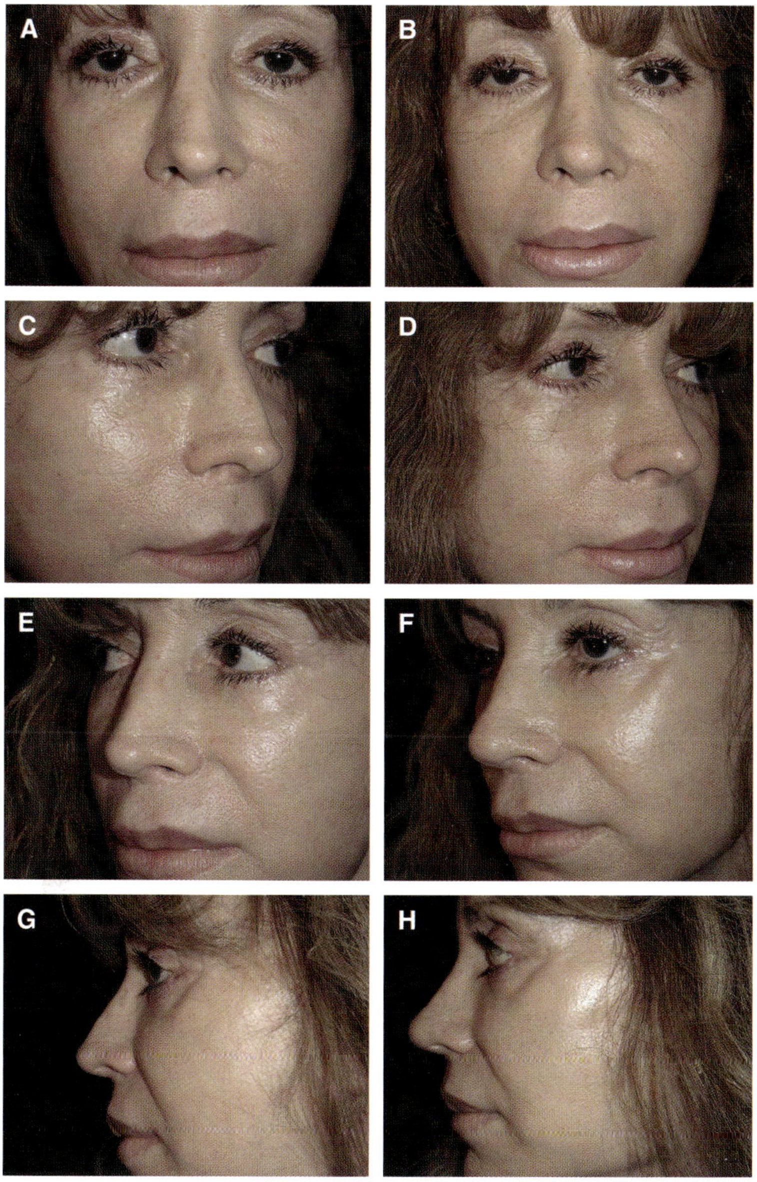

Fig. 8. Pre- (*A, C, E, G*) and posttreatment photos (*B, D, F, H*) of a 62-year-old woman. As a result of secondary rhinoplasty, lack of tip projection and a subtle convexity of the dorsum were some defects to be corrected. After 0.6 mL of Radiesse, tip projection was provided with improved dorsum appearance.

Mid face with HIV-associated facial lipoatrophy

Facial lipoatrophy likely results in part from infection with HIV and in part from highly active antiretroviral treatment as a consequence of the infection. Fat loss is most notable in the cheeks and can cause severe psychological effects because it can be an identifying stigma of HIV infection [42,43]. Treatment of lipoatrophy of the face, therefore, may provide psychological relief for the patient.

Since free fat injections, as proposed for hemifacial atrophy [44], are not available in these specific patients, Radiesse appears to be a very good treatment option.

Infiltrative anesthesia is suggested. The product must be injected in the deep subcutaneous plane by proceeding with a cross-hatching technique. Depending on the degree of hollowness caused by the absence of fat tissue, volumes may vary from patient to patient. In general, 2 to 5 mL per side is recommended (Fig. 9).

Other areas and combinations of treatments

Facial asymmetries can be corrected depending on the required volume. Images in Fig. 10 show how a chin asymmetry was solved with Radiesse. Evans and coworkers [45] presented a report on nipple projection with Radiesse after failed nipple-areolar

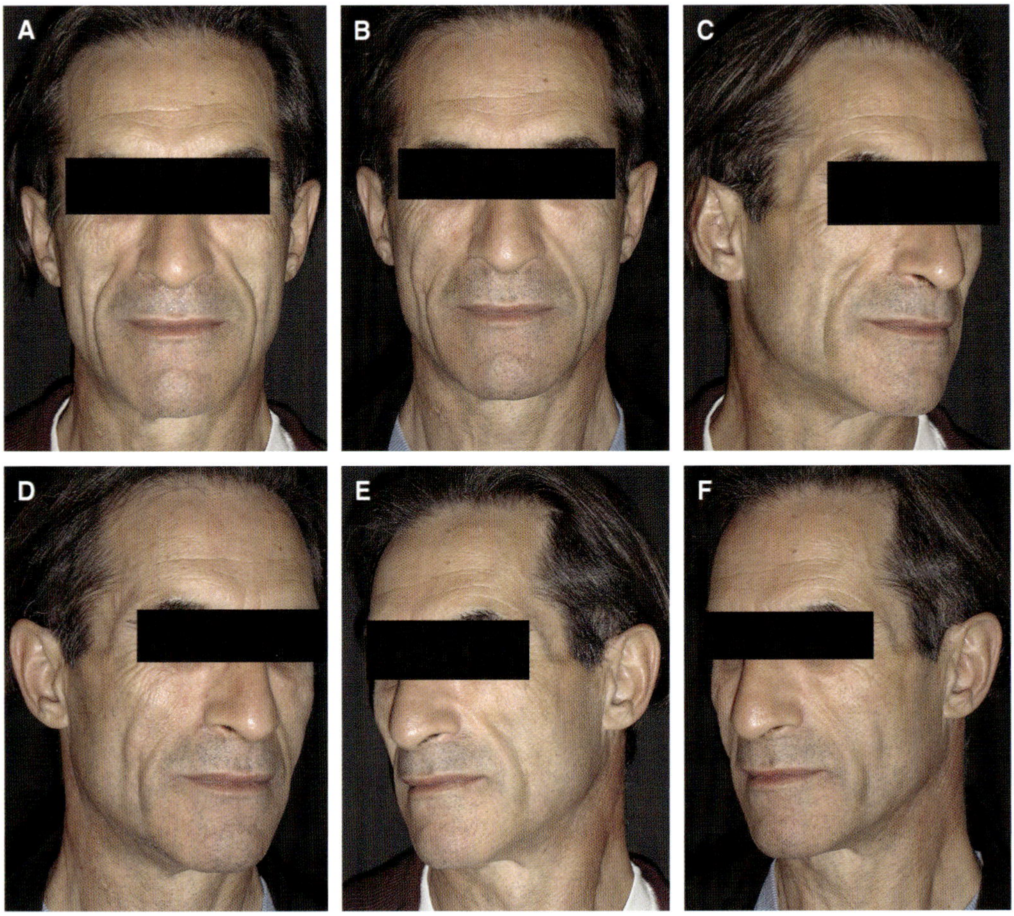

Fig. 9. Pre- (*A, C, E*) and posttreatment photos (*B, D, F*) of a 52-year-old man who had a history of HIV infection since 1990. The patient exhibited extensive facial lipoatrophy and was treated with 3.0 mL of Radiance in the right cheek in 2 sessions and with 2.0 mL in the left cheek. Improvement was accepted as very good after 12 months.

reconstruction. Although the study described early results with only 6 patients, the technique appears to be promising. Godin and colleagues presented an interesting experience with the combination of Radiesse and hyaluronic acid to enhance results in many of the anatomic regions described herein [46].

A preclinical report of effects of monopolar radiofrequency over soft-tissue fillers in an animal model [47] showed an increase in fibroplasia and collagen deposition surrounding Radiesse without harmful consequences.

Botulinum toxin can provide reduction of dynamic wrinkles before Radiesse implant. Proceeding this way, especially in glabellar furrows and marionette lines, filling effects can be improved. Laser treatments, chemical peels and dermabrasion should be performed before a facial filler. As is the case with every patient, variation in circumstance and treatment needs is a given. Each case must be considered as unique according to specific signs, patients' desires, and real possibilities.

Postoperative care

Massaging the treated areas can facilitate even distribution of product. Cold compresses could be applied for first 24 hours on the treated areas. Patients should be aware that the immediate results will regress over the first week after resolution of local edema, and they should be informed that sometimes the implant and the surrounding tissues may be palpable during 30 days after injection. Patients also must be warned that Radiesse may appear on dental x-rays. They should be reminded to tell their dentists about the injection of Radiesse [9].

Results

Patient satisfaction and longevity

In our practice, patient satisfaction results for Radiesse have been followed over an 18-month period. Possible self-reporting options range from very good to good, acceptable and nonacceptable. The

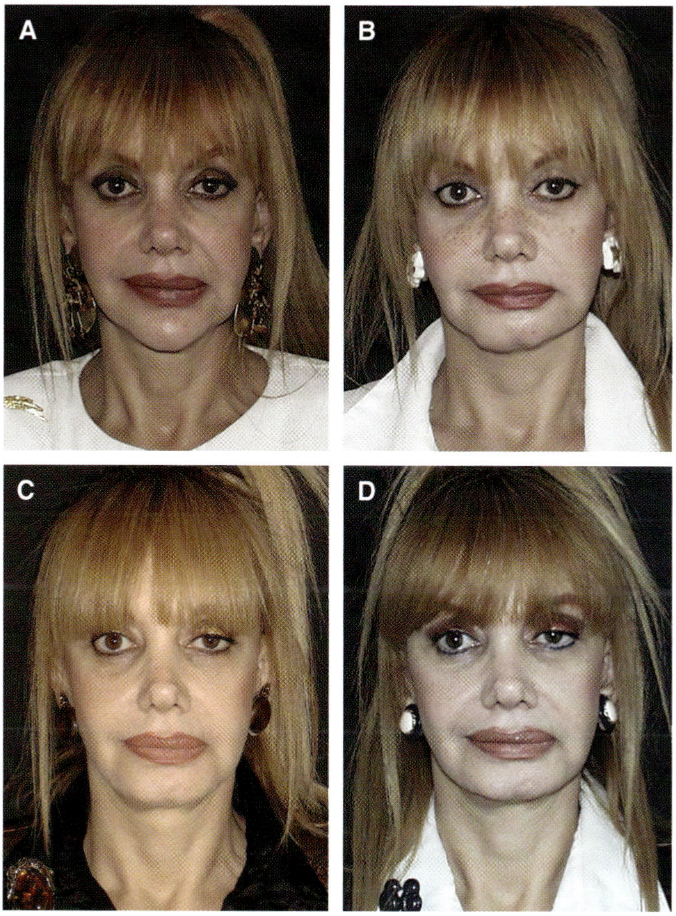

Fig. 10. Sixty-three–year-old woman with asymmetrical displacement of a chin implant (*A*). After chin implant removal, a persistent asymmetry, owing to uneven distribution of natural soft tissue, was her main complaint (*B*). The patient was treated in 2 sessions with 3-months intervals. The images show the results at 12 months (*C*) and at 18 months, after the second touch-up (*D*).

patient self-satisfaction rating for most of the patients (87%) has been very good. No patient has rated the level of satisfaction lower than acceptable. Results achieved during the first postprocedural month and after the last touch-up when needed, remain almost unchanged until 12 months. After 12 to 18 months, the achieved volumes begin to diminish, although some results can be noted 24 months post injection. The average longevity could be considered between 18 and 24 months. Even longer duration of effect can be seen in some patients.

Adverse events and complications

Most of the adverse events and complications associated with soft tissue filler injection are technique related [27]. As temporary adverse effects, ecchymosis and hematoma may be expected in approximately 5% of patients. Some lip nodules have been described as complication [2,10,22,27]. However, these nodules were not granulatomous.

Lip nodules can be treated first with steroid injections and immediate massage. In 50% of the cases, such treatment allows vanishing. Remaining nodules have to be removed surgically through a small incision.

Because asymmetries can occur immediately after injections, the physician should refrain from additional treatment for at least 2 weeks, until the acute inflammatory effects disappear. After that, persistent asymmetries can be corrected. Other adverse effects and complications such as chronic inflammatory reactions, material migration, and difficulty in removal, as reported by Maas [25], have not been seen in this study.

Conclusions

The determination of the appropriate filler material is based on multiple variables. These include patient safety, longevity of effect, surgeons' preferences, and cost-effectiveness ratios. Identifying the many variables before initiating treatment may help with both the decision about which soft tissue filler to use and management of patient expectations of the outcomes and course of treatment. These determinations include precise indications, pitfalls, risks, benefits, advantages, and disadvantages of one soft tissue filler compared with others.

Radiesse has an attractive product profile, for both the patient and the physician. Radiesse requires no allergy tests and is ready for immediate injection. Metabolized through normal phagocytosis, the product has been used in numerous reconstructive surgeries and dentistry for many years. Radiesse has been shown to be biocompatible and an excellent option for the subdermal facial augmentation. The aesthetic effects are immediate, and the injection involves little downtime.

Despite the fact that most of the patients may require a touch-up after 12 months, Radiesse has been fairly predictable, with almost 50% of the initial volume up to more than 24 months in many cases. Compared with short-lasting and permanent products, Radiesse has the advantage of being a long-lasting but not permanent alternative. Nevertheless, through direct and invaluable experience gained over time, plastic surgeons will decide which areas of the face may best be suited for Radiesse and which ones may be appropriate for other fillers.

Acknowledgments

The author thanks David Howell, RRT, and Mariano Meglioli, MD, for the assistance in text and figure processing.

References

[1] Rohrich RJ, Rios JL, Fagien S. Role of new fillers in facial augmentation: a cautious outlook. Plast Reconstr Surg 2003;112:1899–902.

[2] Jansen DA, Graivier MH. Soft tissue substitutes in perioral augmentation. Semin Plast Surg 2003; 17:181–98.

[3] Narins RS, Bowman PH. Injectable skin fillers. Clin Plast Surg 2005;32:151.

[4] Rohrich RJ. Introduction to the Restylane consensus statement. Plast Reconstr Surg 2006; 117(3):1S–2S.

[5] Klein AW, Elson ML. The history of substances for soft tissue augmentation. Dermatol Surg 2000;26:1096–195.

[6] Murray CA, Zloty D, Warshawski L. The evolution of soft tissue fillers in clinical practice. Dematol Clin 2005;23:343–63.

[7] Rohrich RJ, Potter JK. Liquid injectable silicone: is there a role as a cosmetic soft-tissue filler? Plast Reconstr Surg 2004;113:1239–41.

[8] Kanchwala SL, Holloway L, Bucky LP. Reliable soft tissue augmentation. Ann Plast Surg 2005; 55:30–5.

[9] Tzikas TL. Evaluation of the Radiance FN soft tissue filler for facial soft tissue augmentation. Arch Facial Plast Surg 2004;6:234–9.

[10] Carruthers JD et al. Review on long lasting dermal fillers. Medical insight. Available at: www.miinews.com/dermalfillers. Accessed May 25, 2006.

[11] Dover JS. The filler revolution has just begun. Plast Reconstr Surg 2006;117(3S): 38S–40S.

[12] Marmur AS, Phelps R, Goldbeg DJ. Clinical, histologic and electron microscopic findings after injection of a calcium hydroxylapatite filler. J Cosmet Laser Ther 2004;6:223–6.

[13] Havlik RJ and the PSEF Data Committee. Hydroxyapatite. Plast Reconstr Surg 2002;15(4): 1176–9.

[14] Hobar PC, Pantaloni M, Byrd HS. Porous hydroxyapatite granules for alloplastic enhancement of the facial region. Clin Plast Surg 2000; 27(4):557–69.

[15] Bioform Medical Inc. Regulatory issues. Available at: http://www.radiesse.com. Accessed June 12, 2006.

[16] Flaharty P. Radiance. Facial Plast Surg 2000; 20(2):165–9.

[17] Misiek D, Kent J. Soft tissue response to hydroxylapatite particle of different shapes. J Oral Maxillofac Surg 1984;42:150–60.

[18] Pettis G, Kaban L, Glowacki J. Tissue response to composite ceramic hydroxylapatite-demineralized bone implant. J Oral Maxillofac Surg 1990; 48:1068–74.

[19] Probeck HP, Rothstein SS. Histologic observation of soft tissue responses to imported multifaceted particles and discs of hydroxylapatite. J Oral Maxillofac Surg 1989;42:143–9.

[20] Sklar JA, White SM. Radiance FN: a new soft tissue filler. Dermatol Surg 2004;30:764.

[21] Mayer R, Lightfoot M, Jung T. Preliminary evaluation of calcium hydroxylapatite as a transurethral bulking agent for stress urinary incontinence. Urology 2001;57:434–8.

[22] Zide BM. Radiance: short-tern experience. Aesthetic Surg J 2003;23(6):495–9.

[23] Gmyrek R, Dahdah M. Local anesthesia and regional block anesthesia. eMedicine.com. Available at: http://www.emediciene.com/derm. Updated, Jan 19, 2006. Accessed May 25, 2006.

[24] Hanke WC, Higley HR, Jolivette DM, et al. Abscess formation and local necrosis after treatment with Zyderm or Zyplast collagen implant. J Am Acad Dermatol 1991;25:319–26.

[25] Maas CS, Papel ID, Greene D, et al. Complications of injectable synthetic polymers in facial augmentation. Dermatolo Surg 1997; 23:871–7.

[26] Schanz D, Schippert W, Ulmer A, et al. Arterial embolization caused by injection of hyaluronic acid. Br J Dermatol 2002;146:928.

[27] Sclafani AP. Soft tissue fillers for management of the aging perioral complex. Facial Plast Surg 2005;21:74.

[28] Zide BA, Bradley JP, Longaker MT. Lip service for the stiff upper lip. Plast Reconstr Surg 2000;105: 1154.

[29] Guerrissi J. An approach to the senile upper lip. Plast Reconstr Surg 1993;92:1187.
[30] Leaf N, Firous JS. Lip augmentation with superficial musculoaponeurotic system graft, report of 103 cases. Plast Reconstr Surg 2002; 109:319–26.
[31] Linder RM. Permanent lip augmentation employing polytetrafluorowthylene grafts. Plast Reconstr Surg 1992;90(6):1083–90.
[32] Chajchir A, Benzaquen I. Fat grafting injection for soft tissue augmentation. Plast Reconstr Surg 1984;84:921–34.
[33] Nishimura T, Hashimoto H. Microvascular angiogenesis and apoptosis in the survival fat grafts. Laryngoscope 2000;110:1333–7.
[34] Taub PJ, Silver L, Weinberg H. Plastic surgical perspective on vascular endothelial growth factor as gene therapy for angiogenesis. Plast Reconstr Surg 2000;105:1034.
[35] Spira M, Rosen T. Injectable soft tissue substitutes. Clin Plast Surg 1993;20:181–8.
[36] Ersek RA. More on Bioplastique. Aesthetic Plast Surg 2000;24:461.
[37] Lemperle G, Romano JJ, Busso M. Soft tissue augmentation with Artecoll: 10-year history, indications, techniques and complications. Dermatol Surg 2003;29:573.
[38] Honigman RJ, Phillips KA, Castle DJ. A review of psychosocial outcomes for patients seeking cosmetic surgery. Plast Reconstr Surg 2000; 113(4):1229–37.
[39] Dingman RO, Navig P. Surgical anatomy in aesthetic and corrective rhinoplasty. Clin Plast Surg 1977;4:111–20.
[40] Edgerton MT. The art of surgical technique. Baltimore: Williams and Wilkins; 1988.
[41] Gryskiewicz JM. Waste not, want not: the use of Allo Derm in secondary rhinoplasty. Plast Reconstr Surg 2005;116:1999–2004.
[42] James J, Carruthers A, Carruthers J. HIV-associated facial lipoatrophy. Dermatol Surg 2002; 28(11):979.
[43] Comite SL, Liu JF, Balasubramanian S, et al. Treatment of HIV-associated facial lipoatrophy with Radiance FN™ (Radiesse™). Dermatology Online Journal 2004;10(2):2. Available at: http://dermatology.cdlb.org. Accessed May 25, 2006.
[44] Moscona R, Ullman Y, Har-Shay Y. Free fat injection for the correction of hemifacial atrophy. Plast Reconstr Surg 1989;85:508–9.
[45] Evans KK, Rasko Y, Lenert J, et al. The use of calcium hydroxylapatite for nipple projection after failed nipple-areolar reconstruction. Ann Plast Surg 2005;55:25–9.
[46] Godin MS, Majmundar MV, Chrzanowski DS, et al. Use of Radiesse in combination with Restylane for facial augmentation. Arch Facial Plast Surg 2006;8:92–7.
[47] Shumaker PR, et al. Effect of monopolar RF treatment over soft-tissue fillers on an animal model. Laser Surg Med 2006;38(3):211–7.

ELSEVIER
SAUNDERS

CLINICS IN PLASTIC SURGERY

Clin Plastic Surg 33 (2006) 525–538

Hyaluronic Acids

Trevor Born, MD, FRCS(C)

Hyaluronic acid (HA) is a natural substance (complex sugar) found in all living organisms. It hydrates the skin by holding in water, and acts as a cushion and lubricant to reduce damage to the skin. It is found in connective tissue throughout the body, including the dermis. It binds water and gives the tissue its turgor. HAs (in their early formulations) had been used for decades in the United States for intra-articular joint injections and for intraocular treatments [1].

To maintain its presence in the tissue, the HA is cross-linked by various techniques. It is an important component of youthful, supple, and elastic skin, and helps to maintain skin volume. As we age, our skin loses HA, contributing to the formation of wrinkles. Some advantages of the HAs as a group are shown in Box 1.

With the new formulations, the HAs are the most versatile facial/soft tissue fillers on the market. Since the approval of the Restylane family in Canada in 1998 and the approval of Restylane and Hylaform in the United States in 2003 for injection of the nasolabial folds, applications for facial contouring have been varied, with predictable and outstanding results. Numerous publications on techniques support their safety, durability, longevity, and application to reconstructive and cosmetic procedures for both surgical and nonsurgical applications. The incidence of complications is low, and the treatment of complications is relatively straightforward with the use of hyaluronidase. This article discusses the uses of HAs in general, with regard to the various types; Restylane, Captique and Hylaform (available in the United States), and Restylane Fine Lines, Perlane, and Juvederm 18, 24, 30, which are available in Canada and will be available in the United States in the fall of 2006.

In many ways, HAs are the ideal filler. They contain no (or minimal) animal proteins; most are produced with recombinant bacterial technology (except for Hylaform); the longevity allows for a good term of correction without the complications of the longer-lasting fillers (and as other parts of the face age, the corrected areas do not look out of

199 Avenue Road, Suite B, Toronto, Ontario M5R 2J3, Canada
E-mail address: trevor@drborn.ca

0094-1298/06/$ – see front matter
doi:10.1016/j.cps.2006.09.005
plasticsurgery.theclinics.com

Box 1: Advantages of hyaluronic acids

- Relative technical ease to learn and use
- Low incidence of complications
- Multiple areas of use
- Immediate correction with minimal downtime
- Ability to be combined with other therapeutic modalities
- Ease of storage
- Rapid elimination of product with hyaluronidase
- Ability to be repeated
- Minimal long-term effect if therapy is stopped
- Combination effect with Botox
- No known toxic effect
- Relative small needle size for delivery, lessening complications and recovery time

place); they an be combined with other fillers such as ArteFill; they can be placed at all levels of tissue, including right on the periosteum, right on cartilage, and in the mid- to superficial dermis, next to implants such as silicone and polytetrafluoroethylene (PTFE); and they can be layered, using differing particle sizes to achieve maximum change or correction. HAs can be used as a trial for other procedures that may be permanent, such as implants or microfat grafting.

The initial focus of the HAs' use was in the correction of folds, such as the nasolabial, glabellar, and chin fold. Newer uses were described involving restoration of facial volume; reversal of age-related signs in the hands; correction of traumatic deformities of the face and nose; acne scarring; and other adjunctive techniques, such as nipple and earlobe augmentation. The newer HAs (soon to be released) focus on very superficial lines and deep tissue contouring, such as cheek and chin or jaw line augmentation, so that virtually any type of deformity or contour can be changed to achieve the desired result with an HA or a combination of various particle sizes. The newest HA is Restylane Sub Q, which is currently in Food and Drug Administration (FDA) trials. A specific list of the uses of HAs is given in Box 2.

Box 2: Uses of hyaluronic acids

In the face

- Correction of the supraorbital hollows (this is done similarly to the "nonsurgical eyelift") (Airan and Born, personal communication, 2006)
- Correction of the periorbital hollow, or nonsurgical eyelift [2]
- Elevation of the medial eyebrows (personal communication)
- Elevation of the eyebrow; enhancement of eyebrow volume and shape [3]
- Correction of the melomental hollow
- Cheek augmentation
- Chin augmentation
- Correction of nasal deformity: alar, columella, tip, radix, and dorsum
- Acne scar correction
- Lip contouring
- Correction of the mental fold (chin fold)
- Elevation of the corners of the mouth
- Volume augmentation of the posterior jaw line (very useful postfacelift with an aggressive superficial musculatory aponeurotic system (SMAS) and thin skin flap from the neck that leaves the posterior jaw line distorted)
- Augmentation of the inframalar hollow
- Correction of horizontal neck lines
- HIV-associated lipoatrophy
- Correction of deformities associated with endoscopic brow lifts, facelifts, blepharoplasties, suture lifts, and liposuction

Off the face

- Rejuvenation of the hands
- Less commonly performed indications such as earlobe enlargement, nipple enlargement
- Genital contouring

Captique

Captique is a stabilized, HA-based, nonanimal filler. It is indicated for correction of moderate to severe facial wrinkles and folds, such as nasolabial folds. Captique is injected at the level of the deep dermis. It can be used for correction in many different areas of the face, such as nasolabial folds (smile lines), vertical lip lines, marionette lines (lip corners), and crow's feet. The result is reliable and predictable; the longevity varies, but is around 3 months.

Captique was approved in the United States by the FDA in December 2004. Little published data on this product is available. It has the usual side effects associated with dermal fillers, such as redness, bruising, swelling, pain, and itching. Usually, touch-up injections two to three times a year are needed to maintain the correction.

Complications associated with fillers include:

- **Infection**
- **Delayed and immediate hypersensitivity** [5]
- **Uncommon reactions presenting as infection with no response to treatment**
- **Telangiectasia**
- **Tissue necrosis of the nose, glabella, and lip** (Fig. 1) [6]
- **Retinal artery occlusion** [7]
- **Herpetic flare ups**

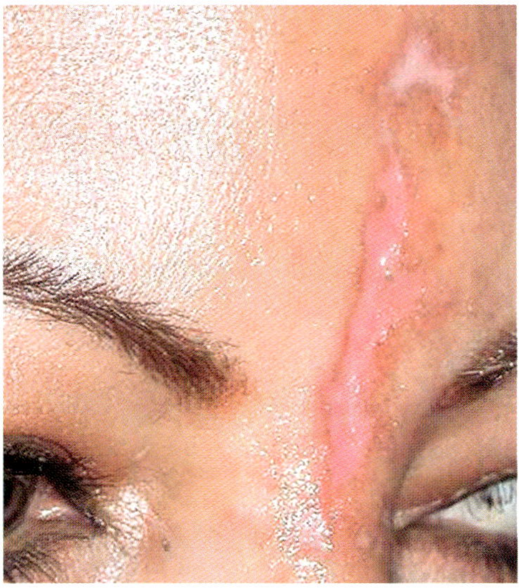

Fig. 1. Necrosis of the glabella postinjection with HA, which resolved without sequelae.

- **Irregularity**
- **Tyndall effect (the product is too close to the epidermis)**
- **Rare cases of systemic symptoms but no documentation as to the specific reaction (Trevor M. Born, personal communication, 2004).**

The Restylane family

The three products available from Q-Med in Sweden are Perlane, Restylane, and Restylane Fine Lines. (These products are also distributed by Medicis in the United States.) They are composed of HA, but differ from each other in their molecular size. Perlane is the largest hyaluronan and Restylane Fine Lines is the smallest. Indications for use depend on size. Perlane is injected at the deepest level in the deep dermis; Restylane is injected in the mid-dermis and the needle should not be visible; and Restylane Fine Lines is injected at the dermoepidermal junction for the most superficial lines. They are 1% cross-linked, are produced by a streptococcal fermentation process, and are referred to as nonanimal stabilized HAs (NASHAs). Restylane contains 100,000 particles per milliliter (mL), Perlane 10,000/mL and Restylane Fine Lines 200,000/mL. The product undergoes isovolemic degradation, so that it absorbs more water as it breaks down, maintaining an equivalent volume over time.

Restylane has been shown to have better longevity than Zyplast [1], and thus a documented [4] better longevity than Hylaform, which showed equivalence to Zyplast in the FDA trial.

Inamed has products that are similar to those offered by Q-Med. Hylaform Plus, Hylaform, and Hylaform Fine Lines are analogous to the Q-Med products and have similar indications. Hylaform Plus is placed in the deep dermis, Hylaform in the mid-dermis, and Hylaform Fine Lines at the dermoepidermal junction. Inamed also owns the rights to Juvederm (Plus), which is another HA product. Juvederm has three sizes as well, Juvederm 30, Juvederm 24, and Juvederm 18, with similar indications to the Restylane family and Hylaform (and Hylaform Plus and Fine Lines as of October 2004) are the only FDA-approved HA fillers in the United States. Perlane and Restylane Fine Lines (or Touch) and the Juvederm family are awaiting FDA approval.

Lip augmentation

Lips can be contoured using many techniques. The technique depends on the patient's goals, the lip shape, and the characteristics of the patient's dentition. The lip with the ideal shape before augmentation will get the ideal result with HAs. Qualities of the lips (upper and lower) that need to be assessed are

- **The length of the upper lip relative to the upper arch (if there is no dental show, then the augmented lip will appear duck-like and too large, especially when the patient smiles)**
- **The length of the philtral columns/upper lip (this needs to be augmented with caution; if the philtral columns are long, then adding volume to them will lengthen the upper lip and detract from the result)**
- **The degree of tightness of the upper lip on the upper dental arch (the tighter the lip is resting on the teeth, the further forward it will project and look more duck-like)**
- **The position of the upper lip relative to the lower lip (ie, occlusion)**
- **The lip thickness (very thin and wide lips can be difficult to add shape to and to contour, and the product tends to disappear very quickly; adding even small volumes can make the lips look unusual or "ducky")**
- **Lesions, scarring; pre-existing irregularity, asymmetry (one side will be longer and the other side will be larger in thickness)**
- **History of herpetic lesions (prophylaxis is necessary)**
- **Dentition (this can be very different between sides of the dental arch; a prominent canine can make the lip look asymmetric)**
- **Other factors, including the patient's age, sex, and profession, all of which relate to the appropriateness of the change in shape desired and to be produced**

The longevity of HAs in the lips is variable. On average, the changes last 4 to 6 months. In general, patients who have very thin lips, broad smiles, or who have very dynamic and mobile lips, will have shorter longevity of the filler (Figs. 2 and 3). Patients who have a more ideal shape and less mobile lips will have better longevity (Figs. 4 and 5). Some individuals may have results that last up to 2 years, and some only 3 months. In some cases, repeat injections may not require the same volume as initial injections. However, individuals get used to the larger volume ("I liked my lips when they were swollen right after the injection") and may want more volume than was done previously. At this point, it is a judgment call in terms of additional volume/size so that the patient's lips are not overdone. The patients who have small or thin lips may have better results and be able to be given more volume on subsequent injections.

Good photographs of the lips should be taken prior, with the mouth in a relaxed, open position in the anterior/posterior and oblique views. These photographs are helpful in documenting pre-existing irregularities and asymmetries.

After the injection, swelling may persist for 3 to 5 days, and there can be bruising for up to 10 days. Any irregularities should be assessed by 1 to 2 weeks, and manual massage should be done to remove them.

Injection technique and level of placement

When Restylane is used for lip augmentation, the injection process generally starts with augmentation of the vermilion border of the lip to enhance its definition and to provide increased projection. The philtral columns may also be augmented; the placement of Restylane at this level is usually in the mid-dermal level. For the vermilion border, placement is along the pseudo-tunnel of the lip border. Caution with the Cupid's bow must be taken with a prominent upper lip; the pseudo-tunnel should be occluded so that the Cupid's bow is not made more prominent. Restylane must not be placed too superficially because it will appear as a light blue color from the Tyndall effect. Palpation of the tissue as the Restylane is injected is important. Occasionally, it can track in a direction perpendicular to the direction of injection because of weakness in the tissue and the vertical lip lines. If this occurs, the Restylane needs to be massaged immediately to eliminate this irregular contour.

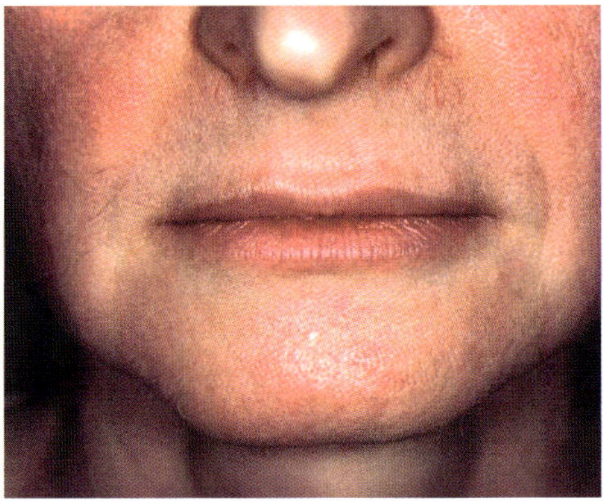

Fig. 3. This patient was injected with 1.0 mL Restylane.

Injection of the lip proper from the wet-dry junction to the vermilion border may also be performed at a level that is just deep to the mucosa within the orbicularis oris muscle. If it is placed immediately beneath the mucosa, then it will be seen as a blue color. Placement posterior to the wet-dry junction along the wet mucosa may enhance the lip volume as well as the projection. Variations in the placement of the product depend on the desires of the patient and the starting shape of the lips. Care must also be taken to observe any previous asymmetries at rest and in animation, scars, weakness, herpetic

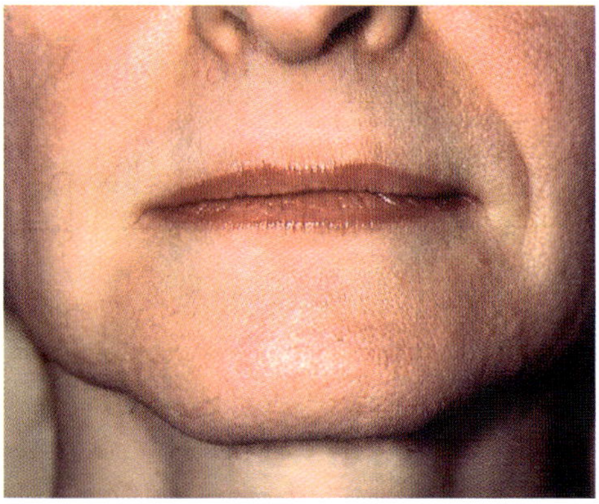

Fig. 2. Example of long thin lips that do not do as well with augmentation.

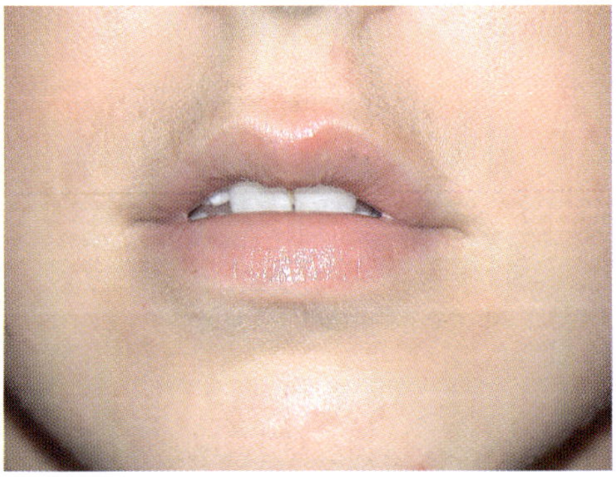

Fig. 4. This patient has ideal lips for augmentation with HAs.

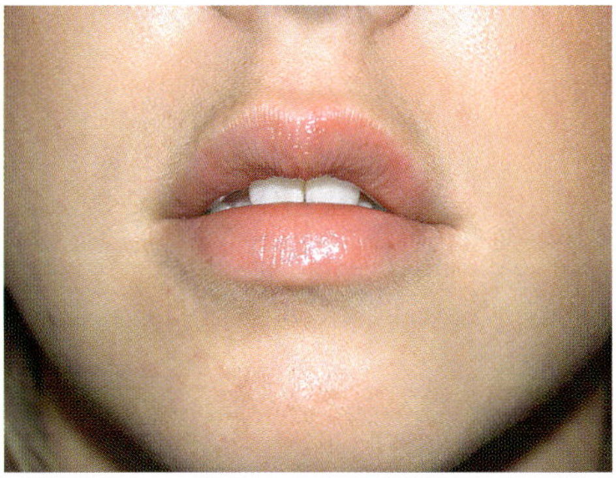

Fig. 5. One month after injection of 1.0 mL Restylane to lips.

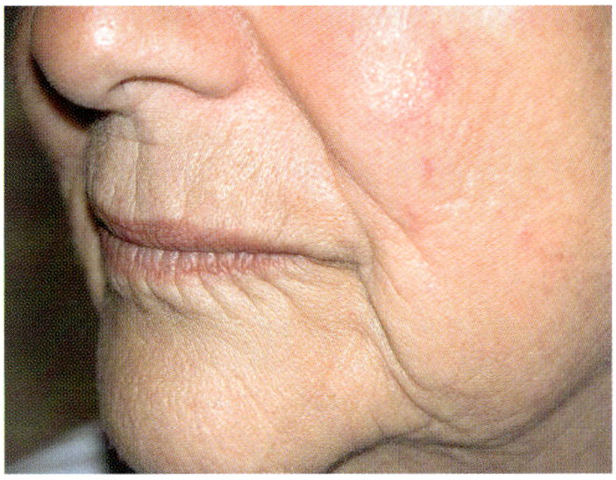

Fig. 6. Atrophy of upper lip above vermillion.

infections, the dentition (including occlusal classification), the length of the philtral column and upper lip, the width of the Cupid's bow, and the depth of the mental fold, all of which can affect the results. Patients who have long thin lips may get limited results due to the tissue tension. Lips that are tight to the dentition or a class II occlusion should be augmented with conservative volumes because the irregularities of the dentition may be reflected in the shape of the lips, making the upper lip appear too prominent or ducky. Scars may not respond to the volume addition and may leave an irregularity. The Cupid's bow becomes wider with age and should be made narrower. The depth of the mental fold increases with age, and softening it can add to the result of the lip contour and improve the overall results of the treatment. Patients who have a prior history of herpes should take prophylaxis; the treatment may cause a herpetic outbreak and scarring.

Frequently, the upper lip is atrophied above the vermilion border, particularly the lateral aspects, and restoration is done with Restylane placed at the mid-dermal level to improve volume and projection of the upper lip here (Fig. 6). This area tends to be a little more vascular, and care should be taken to apply pressure if bleeding is noted. One should use minimal volume in the upper lip above the vermilion border because any added volume may cause lengthening of the upper lip. Care must also be taken to limit the amount of filler placed in the upper lip skin adjacent to the nasolabial fold because this will result in an awkward animation of the upper lip and nasolabial fold, particularly when smiling, and can give the appearance of a joker-type upper lip.

Combined treatment

Some individuals combine Restylane with other tissue fillers. Collagen may be injected first along the vermillion border to provide local anesthesia and augmentation of the white roll. Restylane Fine Lines may be also be used to enhance the white roll; however, Restylane itself works very well in this area. The individual vertical lines of the lips may be corrected with Restylane Fine Lines or collagen.

Restylane can also be used with botulinum toxin type A (Botox). In this situation, Botox may be used in the upper and lower lip orbicularis oris muscle to limit the pinching of the lip and the formation of vertical lip lines. The amount of Botox varies, starting with two units per side of the upper lip avoiding the midline, up to three to four units per side of the upper and lower lip. Rarely, post-Botox in the upper lip, patients have difficulty with pronunciations of Ps and Bs, and difficulty drinking through a straw or out of a cup. If this occurs, the patient may do active puckering of the lips for 15 minutes at a time, several times a day, which will help alleviate these symptoms. Botox will help improve the longevity of the Restylane in the lips and will help to increase lip projection and shape. The Botox may be placed at the vermilion border to a distance of approximately 5 mm away. It must not be placed too far away from the vermillion border because this will result in lengthening of the upper lip and poor shape. The closer Botox is placed to the vermilion border, the greater the lip projection and lip show (red lip).

It is important that good hemostasis with pressure on bleeding points be taken while injecting, so that the lips are not distorted with hematoma, and to prevent vascular complications, such as necrosis of the lip. It is helpful to have a routine approach for every patient so that maximum aesthetic contour can be achieved.

Volumes for lips

Approximate volumes for augmentation of each lip is anywhere from 0.5 to 1.0 mL with Restylane for a total volume of 1 to 2 mL. If Restylane Fine Lines is used 0.5 mL is usually sufficient for the vertical lip lines. Perlane is indicated for lips with good shape for augmentation and are relatively less mobile with similar volumes needed as Restylane. The placement of Restylane in tissue may result in immediate swelling caused by the trauma of needle bruising, or from Restylane absorbing water into its particles and expanding. Immediately postinjection, the lip size should be equivalent to the final result; however, some patients develop swelling caused by bleeding and needle-stimulated histamine release. In the patients who develop immediate swelling, lip shape will be consistent with final results from day 3 to 5. The lips will not increase in size beyond what is placed in terms of volume. If subsequent injections are indicated, then less volume may be required to achieve the desired correction/augmentation, and the lip may be easier to contour (the physician may be able to give more shape and size without the lip looking overcorrected).

Nasolabial folds

As with the lips, the nasolabial folds may be different shapes, lengths, and depths. Some patients have pre-existing telangiectasia, which can be made worse with injections. The gradation system, as described by Dr. Lemperle [8], is useful in evaluating and discussing goals with the patient.

The focus of the correction should be the upper third of the fold, with less emphasis on the lower two thirds of the fold because adding too much filler in this area may be visible with smiling and animation. The amount of change in the average case should be approximately 50% correction of the depth of the fold. Restylane can be used to soften the broader portion of the fold, which is usually the upper two thirds, to the lateral oral commissure. Again, the product is placed at the level of the mid- to deep dermis. Alternatively, Perlane may be used in place of Restylane, and may provide better longevity of the correction. If the nasolabial fold has a superficial line etched into it, this can be softened with Restylane Fine Lines (Figs. 7–10). The product is placed at angles to the fold, and layering may be done to enhance longevity. Perlane may also be placed deep to the Restylane for the very deep folds. With repeated injections of HAs, the product lasts longer and less volume of product is needed to achieve the same volume and contour change. Care must be taken not to overfill the fold because this will give the patient an odd appearance when he/she animates or smiles. Taping the fold for a few days after the injection allows the product to be bound into place with scar tissue, and can prevent the lateral displacement of the product to the nasolabial fold when the patient smiles. Lateral displacement occurs when too much filler is placed, the filler is placed immediately at the margin of the fold, and if the patient has a very broad smile combined with a deep fold and a strong levator labii alaeque nasi.

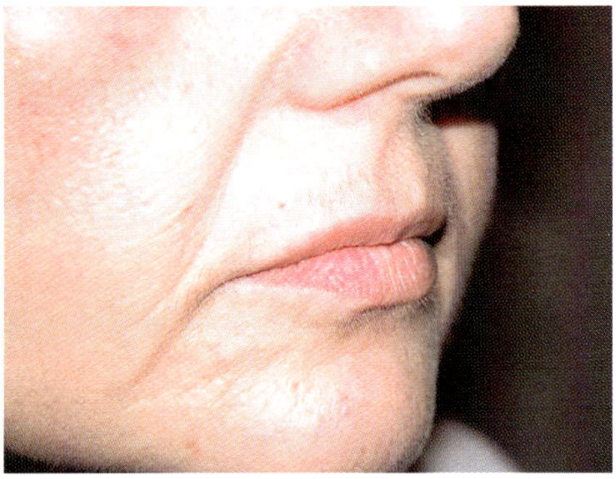

Fig. 7. Preinjection of the nasolabial fold.

Volumes for nasolabial folds

Fold depth is variable. Thus, the amount of filler may range from as little as 0.5 mL to as much as 1.5 mL of Restylane or Perlane. Complete correction of the fold on the first visit is not recommended because this may give the fold an odd appearance. For the first-time treatment, the patient should be instructed that the fold may be corrected by one half of the depth, and further correction will be done at a subsequent injection. This approach has several benefits. It keeps the patient's expectations at a reasonable level; the degree of change is not too drastic; the fold does not feel as firm; it reduces the risk of telangiectasia, which can occur if excessive filler is placed at once; it allows for precise correction of the fold depth and avoids overcorrection of the fold, particularly at the lower one third aspect where it may be over the dentition. The last point is important because if too much dermal filler

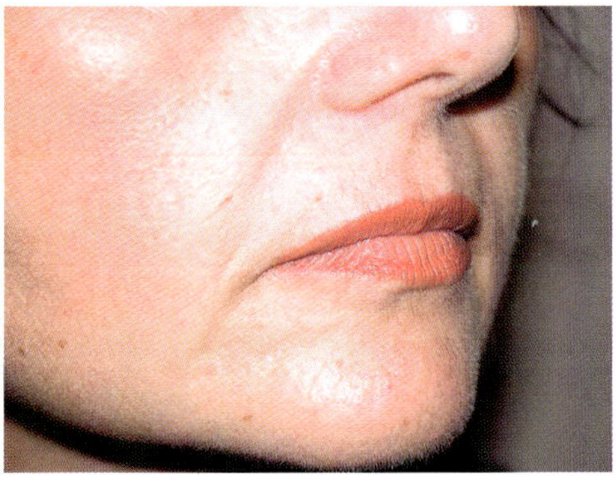

Fig. 8. Six months after injection of 1.1 mL Juvederm.

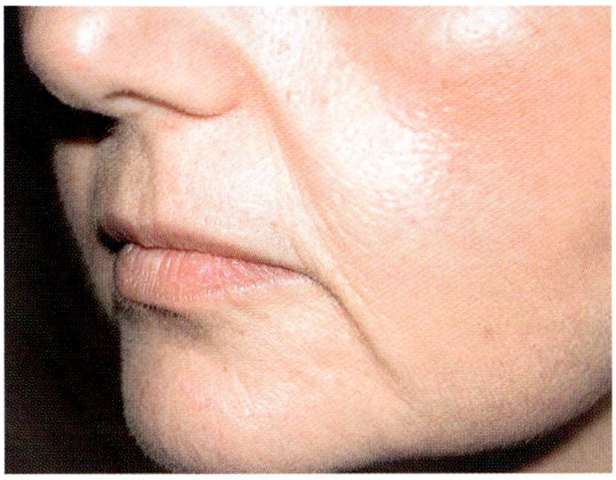

Fig. 9. Preinjection of Restylane to nasolabial fold.

is placed in the fold overlying the dentition, this may appear as a bump, particularly true of the fine but deep marionette lines lateral to the commissure that extend to the melolabial fold.

Scars and deformities

Many deformities of the soft tissue can be corrected with Restylane. It is important that the scar tissue is soft and distensible. The product should not be placed under high pressure because this may result in tissue necrosis. Depth of placement depends a little on the scar characteristics. Generally, the level is the deep dermis; however, the dermis may be thin or atrophic, and thus, deeper placement is required to avoid seeing the filler as a bluish color. Restylane Fine Lines is very effective for small, soft scars such as chicken pox scars. The needle is placed very superficially at the dermal-epidermal junction and a small amount of HA is squeezed into this layer, achieved most easily by placing the needle bevel down (almost parallel to the skin) and barely breaking the skin surface. A small bump may result, but this is then massaged smooth. More than one treatment may be required for full correction.

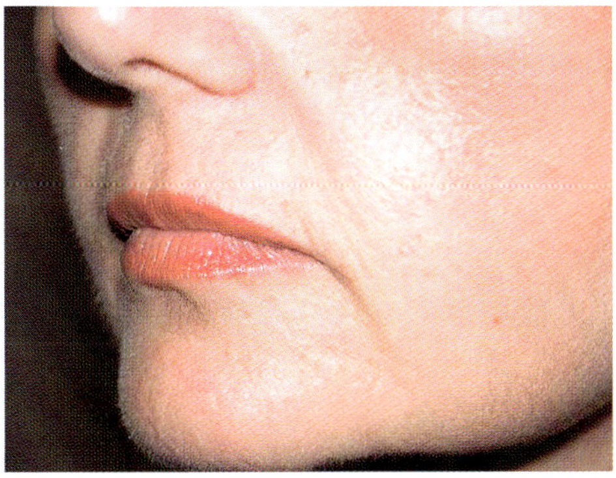

Fig. 10. Six months after injection of 0.75 mL Restylane to nasolabial fold.

Excellent results can be achieved in the nose (post-rhinoplasty deformities), and for acne, chicken pox, and traumatic scars, and the results can be very long lasting. Some release of tissue may be required at the same time, before or after the injection. The use of Restylane Fine Lines in steroid atrophy is helpful, but it must be used with caution because the atrophy may be permanent. The patient should be warned of this so that the HA is not considered the cause of the deformity.

For nasal deformities, the injections may be done at the dermal and subdermal level, depending on the area. In Figs. 11 and 12, the postrhinoplasty deformity has been corrected with 0.5 mL Restylane at the subdermal level.

Volumes for scars and deformities

The volumes may be variable, with very small amounts (less than 0.05 mL) for acne or chicken pox scars placed at a superficial level (dermal-epidermal junction), and up to 0.2 mL for larger soft acne scars placed at the mid- to deep dermis. Layering of the fillers may be needed (Restylane for deep and Restylane Fine Lines for more superficial). The use of Botox in conjunction is helpful for scars located in mobile areas such as the glabella, forehead, and chin, or for lips, where the mimetic action may be reduced. Use of Botox may also increase the longevity of the filler placed.

Glabellar folds

Ideally, the vertical folds of the glabella are treated in combination with Botox [9]. There may be several lines and folds, differing in depth and width.

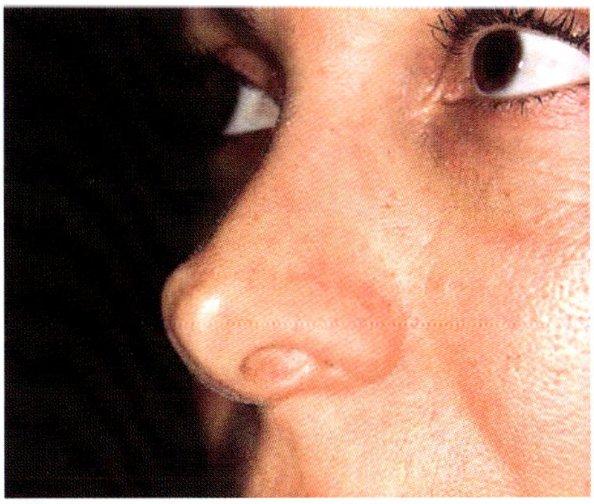

Fig. 11. This patient had a rhinoplasty as a teenager, with a residual nasal tip deformity. This deformity was corrected with 0.5 mL Restylane injected at the subdermal level. The result at 2 years is shown in Fig. 12.

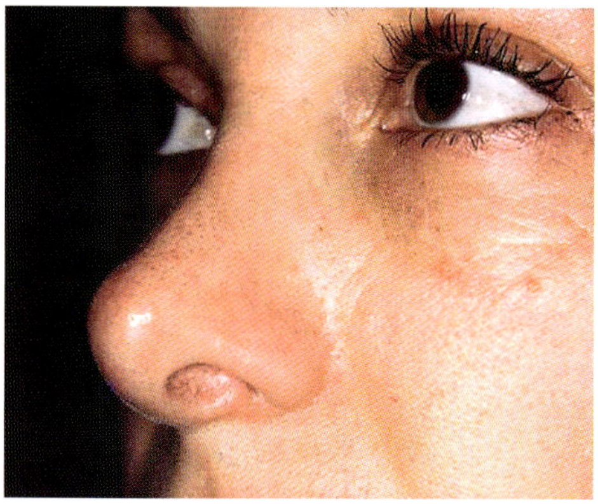

Fig. 12. Post-Restylane 0.5 mL.

If the fold is effaced easily (ie, flatten the fold and it remains soft), Botox may soften the fold on its own. The glabellar fold may be a fairly superficial line with a deeper etched component that is best treated with Restylane Fine Lines at the dermal-epidermal junction; this is placed in a pin-point fashion, with serial linear injections at the same level undermining the line and in a crisscross fashion. If the fold is wide, then Restylane may be placed at the mid-dermis to superficial dermis by a linear threading technique. Small amounts must be injected to avoid tissue necrosis. When combined with Botox, the effect can last from 8 months to being corrected permanently.

Volumes for glabellar folds

A range of 0.25 to 0.5 mL of Restylane and up to 0.5 mL of Restylane Fine Lines may also be needed for correction, depending on the number of folds and their depth.

Brow elevation

Eyebrow elevation with Botox can be enhanced with the HAs. The Carruthers describe their technique with Restylane; the needle is placed in the subdermal plane (at the level of the brow fat pad) at the lateral eyebrow cilia, with the needle at a 45-degree angle. A push-ahead technique is used (ie, the Restylane/HA is injected as the needle is advanced) to inflate the volume, thus raising the eyebrow. This procedure appears to be very effective for the lateral eyebrow and since 2000, by the Carruthers, has had good longevity with no vascular complications. Approximately 0.5 mL is needed in general for each side.

Eyebrow elevation can also be achieved with injection of HA on the layer next to, or under, the periosteum. This method is advantageous because the filler is hidden by multiple layers, lessening the chance of an irregularity being seen or felt. This area is also less mobile, and the filler tends to persist for 8 months to 1.5 years, similar to the treatment of the lower eyelid, as described in the article, "Non-Surgical Eyelift," by Dr. Lisa Airan and the author in 2005 [2].

This technique can help raise both the medial and lateral eyebrow (author's note). If the area is infiltrated directly with local adrenaline, bruising is limited. Restylane in the amount of 0.5 to 1.0 mL per side is used. A modification of this technique can correct the supra-orbital hollow that may be caused by too much fat and skin resection of the upper lid, or by fat atrophy of the periorbital region, associated with aging. It also gives the illusion of raising the eyebrows.

Elevation of the medial eyebrow can also be achieved with the placement of Restylane in the mid- to superficial dermal layer, best done in combination with Botox to weaken the depressors of the medial eyebrow. The Restylane is injected from the radix to the medial aspect of the eyebrow, either by a push technique or linear threading, to increase the stiffness of the skin, thus pushing the medial eyebrow in the superior direction (similar to raising the corner of the mouth described by Dr. Arnie Klein [10]). The above procedures can be combined to give incredible results in upper eyelid and eyebrow shaping. Caution must be taken when injecting in this region.

The hollow lower eyelid: the nonsurgical lower eyelid lift

The lower eyelid may have a hollow appearance that is congenital or a result of aging. The correction of the hollow was described by Drs. Airan and Born in the November 2005 issue of Plastic and Reconstructive Surgery. The basic approach is to fill the depth of the hollow with Restylane on the deep layer next to the bone (at the subperiosteal level) [2].

The area is infiltrated first with local anesthesia and adrenaline to help with hemostasis and to free the deep layer of tissue to allow easy placement of the Restylane. Complete correction of the hollow is performed from the lateral orbital rim to the medial orbital rim, along with correction of the infra malar hollow, if needed. Careful palpation of the infraorbital rim and protection of the globe at all times should be done with the noninjecting hand. Care must be taken not to place the Restylane behind the orbital septum because swelling of the lower lid fat can result; if this happens, 75 units of hyaluronidase in local anesthesia + adrenaline will correct this. The result can last up to 1.5 years and, because it is on the deep layer, irregularity is very uncommon (Figs. 13–16).

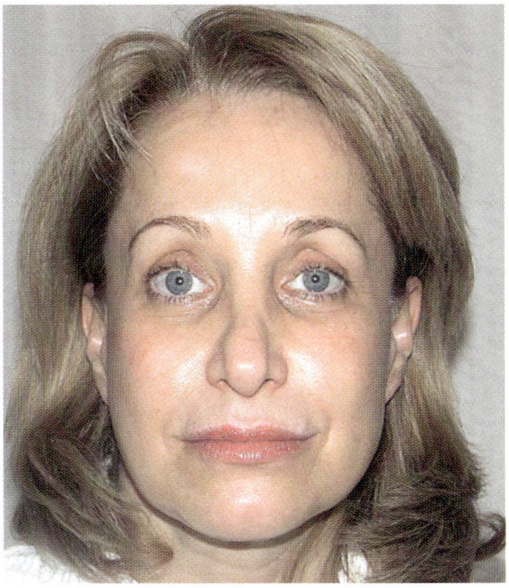

Fig. 13. Pre-Restylane to infraorbital hollow, anterior view and pre-Restylane injection of the lateral brow (on the periosteum).

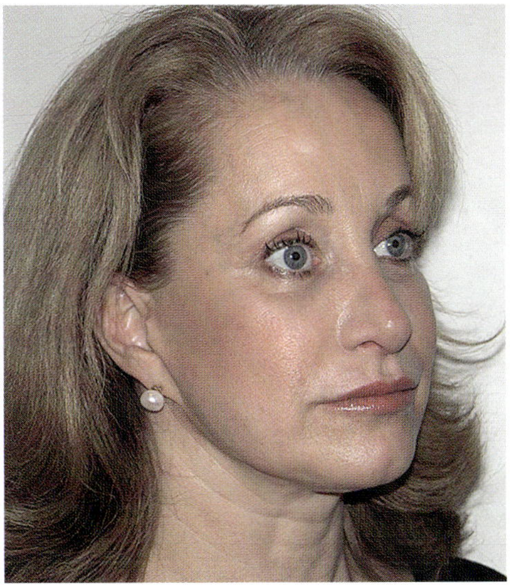

Fig. 15. Preinjection of Restylane into the infraorbital hollow.

Three other techniques have been described. Michael Kane [11] places the Restylane with a 32-gauge needle in the immediate subdermal plane of the lower eyelid. He describes the correction of the hollow and rejuvenation of the eyelid tone and shape. This procedure is performed with multiple passes, with very small amounts of Restylane being placed with each pass to avoid irregularity and to provide an even layer of thickening to the whole lower lid.

Val Lambros describes the correction of the medial orbital hollow with injection of Restylane in the submuscular layer at the deepest point of the hollow, using 0.3 to 0.4 mL per side with good longevity. The Restylane is placed carefully and then massaged with a finger tip to smooth any irregularity.

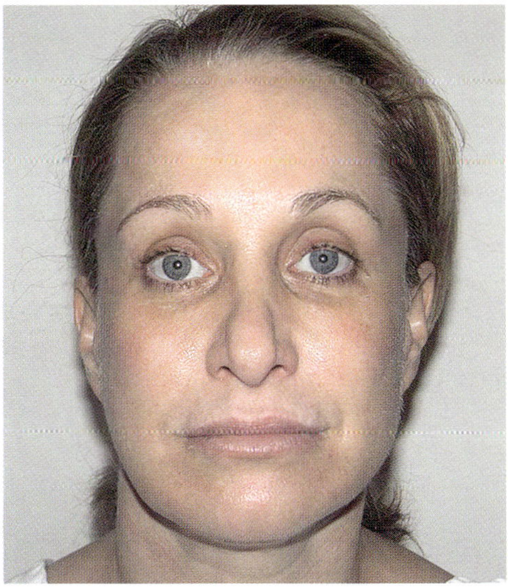

Fig. 14. Postinjection of 1.0 mL Restylane in the infraorbital hollow, giving a nonsurgical eyelift anterior view and elevation of lateral eyebrows with Restylane, 0.5 mL injected beneath the periosteum of the lateral brow.

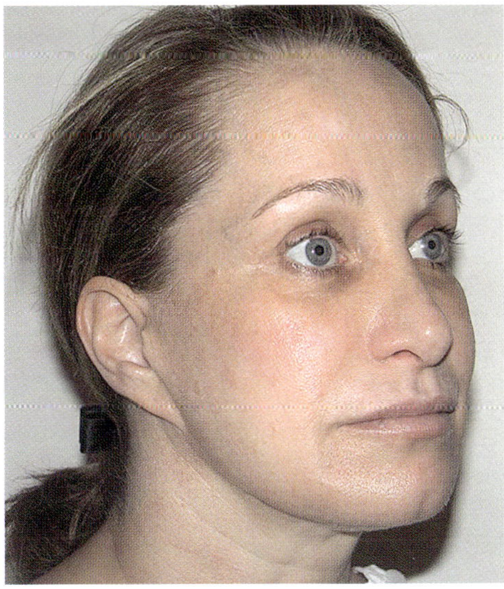

Fig. 16. Postinjection of Restylane into the infraorbital hollow (1.0 mL Restylane per side). Note complete elimination of hollow, which is noted particularly at the lateral aspect of the orbital rim.

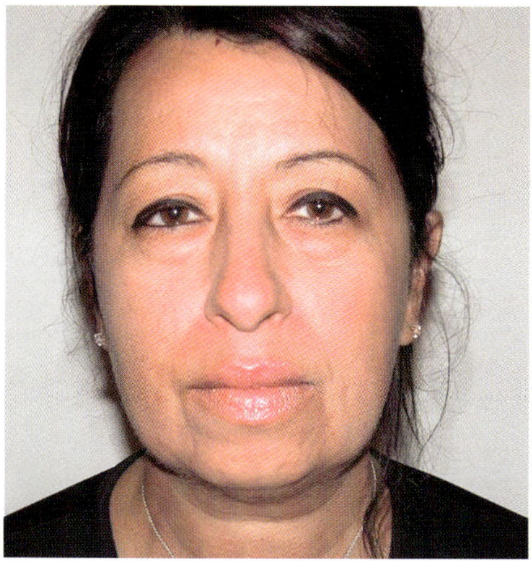

Fig. 17. Preinjection with Restylane Sub Q to cheeks and chin, anterior view.

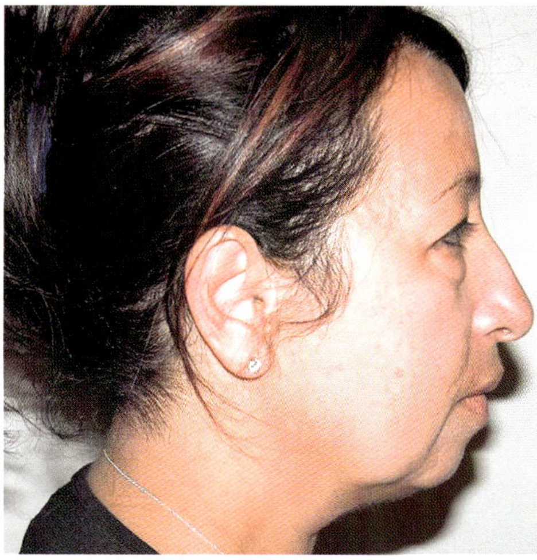

Fig. 19. Preinjection of Restylane Sub Q to cheek and chin, lateral view.

The Carruthers describe the correction of the nasojugal fold with the placement of the filler deep to the orbicularis oculi muscle, just along the periosteum at the arcus marginalis [10]. They use HAs or collagen for their technique.

Cheek augmentation

Cheek volume may be increased by various techniques. The newest is with Restylane Sub Q. This filler, a member of the NASHA family from Q Med, is undergoing FDA trials. The particles are 10 times larger than Perlane and are visibly about 2 mm in length. The product is placed on the deep layer, next to the bone, using an 18-gauge cannula in bolus format and a small transcutaneous incision (an intraoral incision may also be used). Care must be taken not to inject the product while the cannula is withdrawn because the particles will track along the passage of the cannula, become mobile, and form a bump. Augmentation of the malar prominence up to the orbital rim and posterior along the zygomatic arch will give very nice correction/augmentation for up to 12 months or longer (Figs. 17–20). The procedure takes about 15 minutes and requires infiltration of local anesthesia with adrenaline for hemostasis. Complications include infection, irregularity, and temporary infraorbital nerve dysesthesia. The Sub Q may also be used

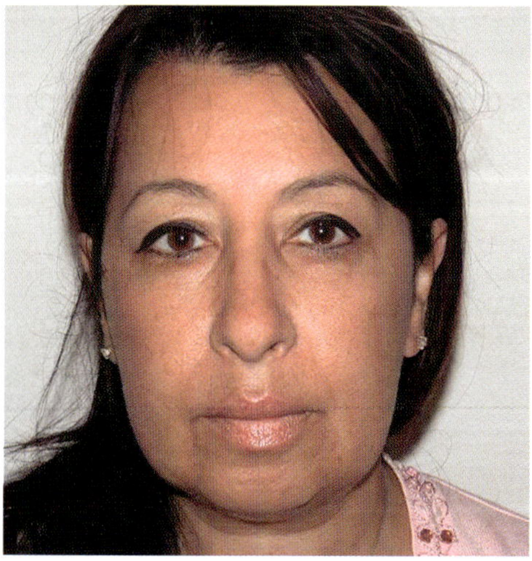

Fig. 18. Postinjection with Restylane Sub Q, 4 mL per cheek. Note increase in cheek projection and masking of the prominent lower eyelid fat; 2.5 mL Restylane Sub Q for chin augmentation is less impressive, but nonetheless a good result.

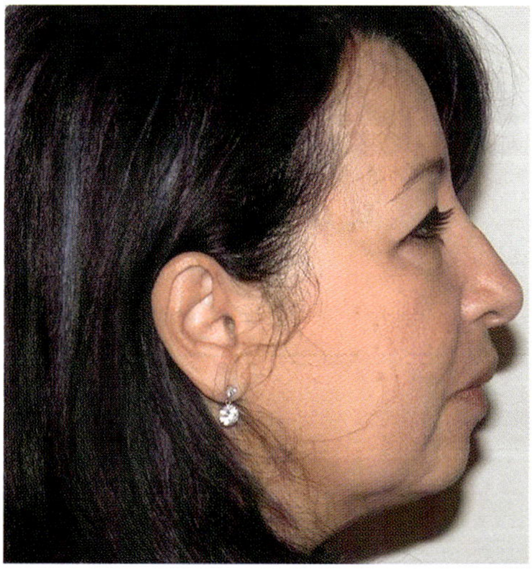

Fig. 20. Postinjection of Restylane Sub Q to cheeks and chin placed on the bony level. Note the significant changes in this view.

in a similar fashion for chin augmentation. In general, 2 to 3 mL per cheek, up to 4 mL, are used.

The cheek may also be augmented in a more subtle fashion with Perlane or Restylane. The filler is placed in the subdermal space in the area requiring augmentation. Care must be taken not to inject the filler into the orbicularis oculi muscle because this may appear as an irregularity. Amounts of 0.5 to 1.0 mL per side or more may be used. Botox may be used to soften the crow's feet, but care should be taken not to weaken the orbicularis oculi muscle too much because it is an elevator of the cheek, and this may increase the hollow of the eye, or deepen the fold created by the zygomaticus major when smiling.

Chin augmentation

The chin may be augmented at both the dermal level and on the deep layer next to the bone. As with cheek augmentation with Restylane Sub Q, one uses the technique of placement with a transcutaneous incision and deposition of the Sub Q on the deep layer beneath the mentalis muscle. Amounts of 1.5 to 2 mL may be used by way of two or three incisions. An increase in projection of 1 mm to 4mm can be achieved.

Perlane in the dermal plane by a push-ahead technique can give more subtle augmentation in both the vertical and anterior/posterior planes. Perlane may be placed on the bone as well, giving similar results to Sub Q. The typical volume required is 0.5 to 1.5 mL. Concomitant use of Botox can improve the results and the longevity of the filler.

The mental fold can become deeper with time, and this can be softened with mid-dermal placement of Restylane. A layer of Restylane Fine Lines may be placed on top of this if the line is etched into the skin. Botox placed into the mentalis muscle will give marked improvement and longevity as well.

Melomental hollow

Loss of volume of the area anterior to the jowl and along the jaw line occurs with aging. By adding volume to this area, the jowl can be disguised and the shape of the jaw line straightened. The correction is done on two levels. The inferior portion along the jaw line and overlying the mandible is corrected at the bony level in a fashion similar to the nonsurgical eyelift. Perlane is injected by placing the needle through the skin, down to the bone and in a bolus technique, providing 75% of the correction with approximately 0.5mL. Next, the remainder of the hollow is corrected by a deep dermal injection of Restylane, using a push-ahead technique, starting at the jaw line and working to the corner of the mouth to provide a pillar support and elevate the corner of the mouth. The deep layer (bone level) injection of Perlane provides good longevity for the correction. This region may bruise more than other areas. Combining the procedure with an injection of Botox into the depressor anguli oris helps improve the longevity of the filler by decreasing the movement of the tissue in this region (Figs. 21 and 22).

Horizontal neck rhytids

Neck rhytids can be softened with injection of Restylane or Restylane Fine Lines at the dermal/epidermal level (with a 32 gauge needle). Botox placed in the platysma will aid in giving an excellent result.

Aging hands

The prominence of the veins and tendinous interspaces are aging signs. Options for correction include microfat grafting, Sculptra, and Restylane injections.

Restylane is placed in the mid-dermal level in very small amounts adjacent to the veins and tendons to provide camouflage. The technique is subtle, and can be difficult in patients who have thinning skin. As the structures in the subcutaneous plane are mobile, care must be taken to place only small amounts of HA over a wider area. The procedure can be performed with topical anesthesia or a dorsal wrist block. Between 1 and 2 mL of Restylane per hand may be required (Figs. 23 and 24).

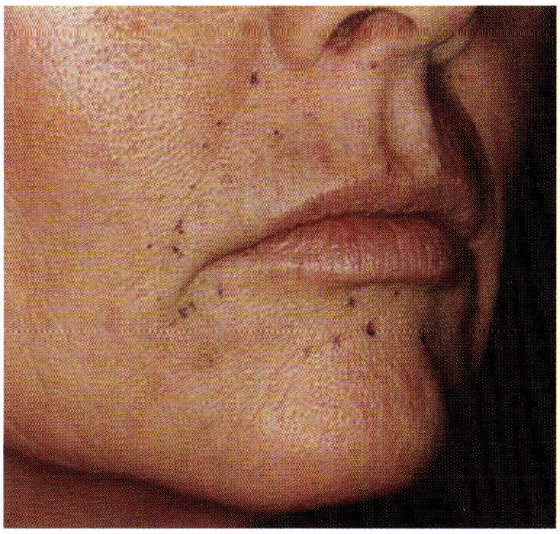

Fig. 21. Oblique view of the melomental hollow before filling with Perlane on the bone layer, Restylane at the deep dermal level, and Restylane Fine Lines for the superficial lines.

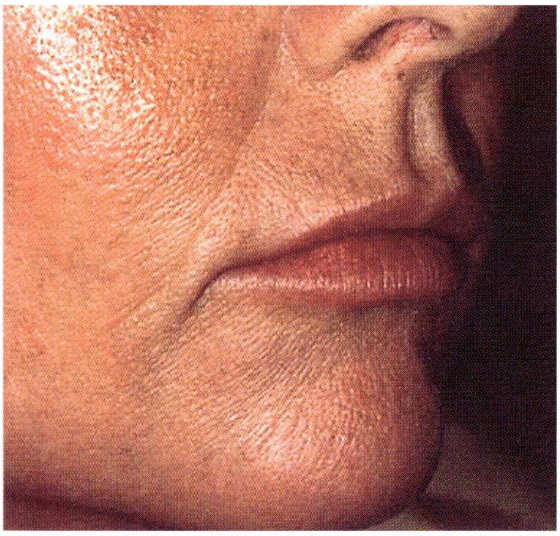

Fig. 22. Postinjection of HAs. Note the overall improvement of contour of the perioral area, softness of the mouth appearance, and the correction of the corner of the mouth.

Combination therapy

HAs can be combined safely with other fillers such as Artecoll/ArteFill, overlying silicone implants, and Sculptra (Danny Vleggaar, MD, personal communication, 2006). The timing depends on the end result desired. Artecoll may be used to set a layer of scar tissue deep, and the HA placed over the top 2 months after Artecoll injection, as in Figs. 25–28.

Longevity

The degree of longevity depends on the metabolism of the individual and the amount of movement with animation. In general, patients who are more animated have a shorter duration of filler. The filler remains in the tissue for up to 16 months, although with diminished intensity. For most individuals, more augmentation may be achieved at secondary and tertiary injections, which build upon the

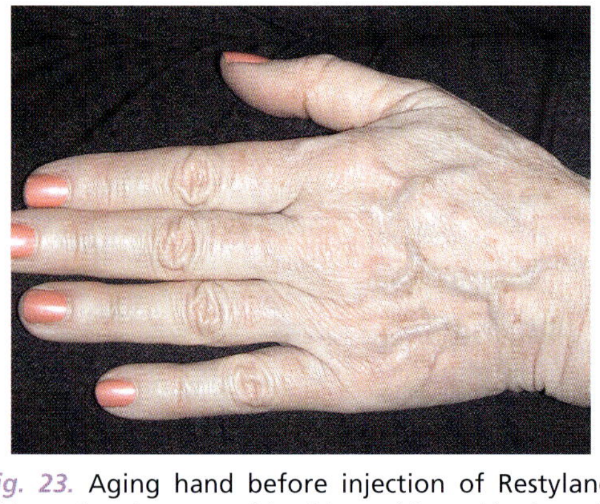

Fig. 23. Aging hand before injection of Restylane. This patient has very thin skin and is an ideal candidate for fat grafting.

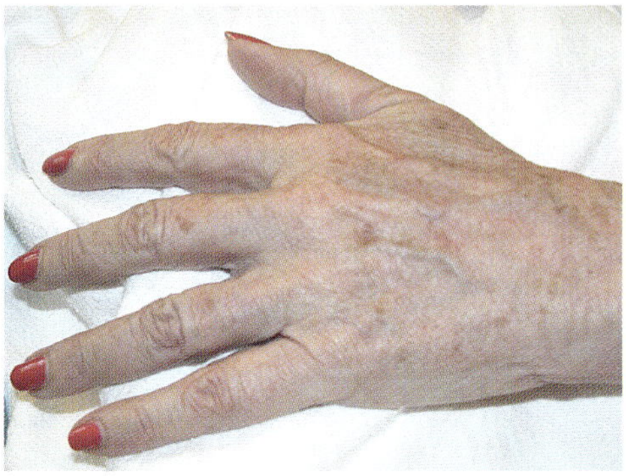

Fig. 24. Postinjection of Restylane to the dorsum of the hand.

remaining filler and allow for further shaping, enhancement of volume, and contouring of the lips when subsequent injections are performed. The filler should last for a period of 4 to 6 months; however, when it is repeated the results may last 8 months to a year. In some individuals, the filler may disappear after as little as 3 months, and may require repeat contouring.

Postinjection care

Immediate postinjection control of swelling and bruising is controlled with antihistamines, coolpacks for 20 minute periods over 24 hours, and massage (only to be performed by the physician or physician instructions). The individual should be seen at 1.5 to 2 weeks after the initial injection to assess for any irregularities, lumps, bumps, or asymmetries. If a bump is discovered, then it may be massaged. If this does not alleviate the irregularity, injection of hyaluronidase may be performed, if available. The dose may be 10 to 15 units injected with local anesthesia and adrenaline to limit the area affected by the enzyme.

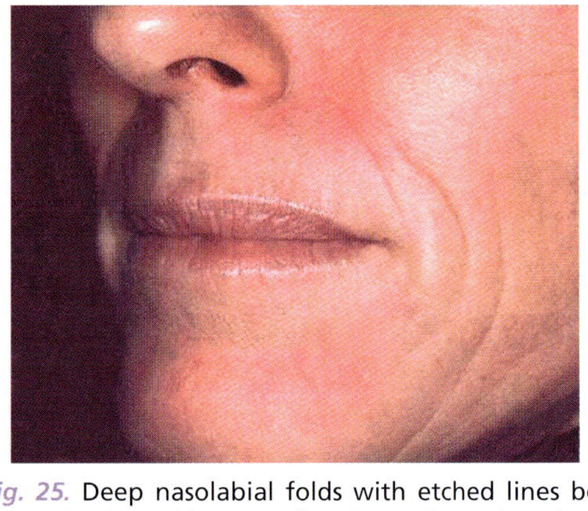

Fig. 25. Deep nasolabial folds with etched lines before injection with Artecoll and Restylane Fine Lines.

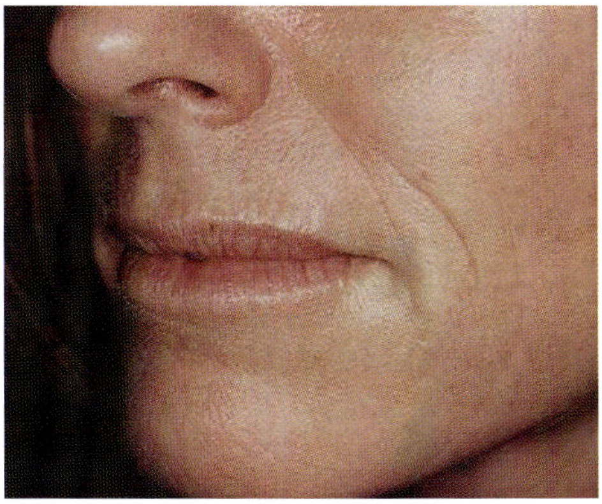

Fig. 26. Artecoll placed on the deep dermal layer to provide support for placement of Restylane Fine Lines, oblique view.

The patient should be informed that swelling will occur in the first 3 to 5 days after injection, which may make the lips appear overdone. This swelling will resolve, but possible bruising could last up to 1.5 weeks.

Persons with long thin lips and very broad smiles are difficult to augment. Care should be taken to provide adequate consultation and the information that the result they desire may not be achievable with one, or even subsequent, injections.

Side effects, reactions, and complications

When larger volumes of filler are used at one time, a sterile abscess requiring drainage may occur up to 1 to 2 weeks after the initial injection. Other complications that may occur are lumps, bumps, irregularities, numbness of the lip, pain, hematoma, and overcorrection. The occasional individual will have massive swelling in response to the injection (caused by the needle or the HA) and one may consider using a Medrol Dose Pack to alleviate this immediate swelling. Risks of steroid use should be explained as well. Postinjection treatment includes cooling with ice packs (20 minutes on and 20 minutes off for the first 24 hours) and oral antihistamines, which may be administered before the treatment (eg, Claritin, Zyrtec, or Allegra in usual daily doses). A rare event of tissue necrosis or ischemic compromise should be treated urgently with a topical vasodilator, such as nitro paste, and injection with hyaluronidase (see Fig. 1).

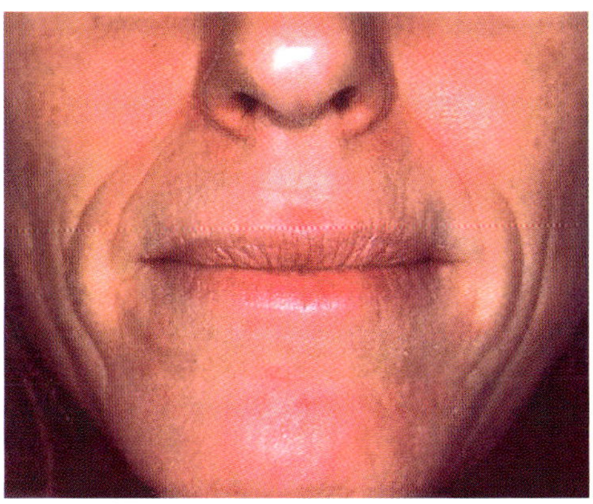

Fig. 27. Pre-Artecoll and Restylane Fine Lines, anterior view.

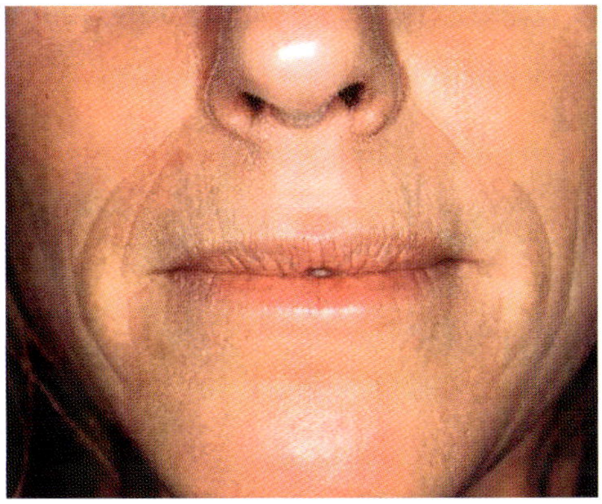

Fig. 28. Post-Artecoll and Restylane Fine Lines.

Further readings

American Society of Plastic Surgeons; American Society for Aesthetic Plastic Surgery. Injectables and fillers: legal and regulatory risk management issues. Plast Reconstr Surg 2006 Sep;118(3 Suppl):129S–132S.

Matarasso SL, Carruthers JD, Jewell ML, Restylane Consensus Group. Consensus recommendations for soft-tissue augmentation with nonanimal stabilized hyaluronic acid (Restylane). Plast Reconstr Surg 2006;117(3 Suppl):3S–34S, discussion 35S-43S.

References

[1] Biesman B. Soft tissue augmentation using Restylane. Facial Plast Surg 2004;20:171.

[2] Plastic and Reconstructive Surgery: Volume 116(6) November 2005 pp 1785–1792

[3] Kornstein AN. Soft-tissue reconstruction of the brow with Restylane. Plast Reconstr Surg 2005; 116(7):2017.

[4] Rao J, Chi GC, Goldman MP. Clinical comparison between two hyaluronic acid-derived fillers in the treatment of nasolabial folds: Hylaform versus Restylane. Dermatol Surg 2005;31(11 Pt 2): 1587.

[5] Matarasso S, Herwick R. Hypersensitivity reaction to nonanimal stabilized hyaluronic acid. J Am Acad Dermatol 2006;55(1):128.

[6] Andre P. Evaluation of the safety of a non-animal stabilized hyaluronic acid (NASHA—Q-Medical, Sweden) in European countries: a retrospective study from 1997 to 2001. J Eur Acad Dermatol Venereol 2004;18:422–5.

[7] Peter S, Mennel S. Retinal branch artery occlusion following injection of hyaluronic acid (Restylane). Clin Experiment Ophthalmol 2006;34(4):363.

[8] Lemperle G, Holmes RE, Cohen SR, et al. A classification of facial wrinkles. Plast Reconstr Surg 2001;108(6):1735–50.

[9] Carruthers J, Carruthers A. A prospective, randomized, parallel group study analyzing the effect of BTX-A (Botox) and nonanimal sourced hyaluronic acid (NASHA, Restylane) in combination compared with NASHA (Restylane) alone in severe glabellar rhytides in adult female subjects: Treatment of severe glabellar rhytides with a hyaluronic acid derivative compared with the derivative and BTX-A. Dermatol Surg 2003; 29:802.

[10] Carruthers J, Klein AW, Carruthers A, et al. Safety and efficacy of nonanimal stabilized hyaluronic acid for improvement of the mouth corners. Dermatol Surg 2005;31:276.

[11] Kane MA. Treatment of tear trough deformity and lower lip bowing with injectable hyaluronic acid. Aesthetic Plast Surg 2005;29(5): 363.

CLINICS IN PLASTIC SURGERY

ELSEVIER SAUNDERS

Clin Plastic Surg 33 (2006) 539–550

Sculptra: the New Three-Dimensional Filler

Richard N. Sherman, MD[a,b]

Sculptra (Dermik Laboratories, A Division of Aventis Pharmaceuticals, Inc., Berwyn, PA) was approved by the US Food and Drug Administration (FDA) on August 3, 2004 as the first synthetic injectable medical device for the treatment of HIV-related facial lipoatrophy [1]. HIV lipodystrophy syndrome is a complication of highly active antiretroviral therapy (HAART) with protease inhibitors (PIs) or nucleoside reverse transcriptase inhibitors (NRTIs) [2–7]. HIV lipodystrophy syndrome is characterized by metabolic abnormalities, central fat hypertrophy, and peripheral fat atrophy. Metabolic aberrations (insulin resistance/diabetes, hypercholesterolemia, and hypertriglyceridemia) and central fat hypertrophy are more commonly seen with PIs, whereas NRTIs are more likely to contribute to fat wasting or lipoatrophy [6]. Metabolic changes may eventually require medication with oral hypoglycemic, antilipid agents, or both.

The phenomenon of abnormal fat distribution, affecting 30% to 80% of patients on HAART, may be a consequence of PIs and NRTIs or may be interpreted as a long-term complication of HIV disease [2,6]. The search for optimal treatment of these abnormal fatty changes continues. Hypertrophic fat deposition occurs most commonly in the truncal area with a predilection for the dorsocervical region (buffalo hump/hoarse collar), lower abdomen (crix belly/protease paunch), and breasts. Although human growth hormone has been demonstrated to improve central obesity of the abdomen, breasts, and buffalo hump, recurrence with cessation of therapy is likely [8]. Localized liposuction of hypertrophic fatty deposits using tumescent anesthesia is safe, effective, and provides cosmetic improvement [9].

Atrophic fatty changes may present as peripheral wasting of the face, extremities, and buttocks.

[a] Skin Institute of New Orleans, 2633 Napoleon Avenue, Suite 815, New Orleans, LA 70115, USA
[b] Department of Dermatology, Tulane University, New Orleans, LA, USA
E-mail address: rshermanmd@cox.net

doi:10.1016/j.cps.2006.09.001
plasticsurgery.theclinics.com

Prolonged duration of antiviral therapy, specific antiviral agents (especially stavudine [Zerit]), combination therapy using PIs and NRTIs, advancing age, low body weight, and incomplete viral suppression contribute to the progression of lipoatrophy [10]. The treatment of the atrophic component of HIV lipodystrophy syndrome represents a therapeutic and cosmetic challenge. Androgens, such as testosterone and nandrolone, may increase muscle mass, enhancing body form and camouflaging lipoatrophy of the extremities [6,11,12]. Chronic steroid use may, however, increase the risk of hepatotoxicity and lead to diabetes, making such treatment regimens controversial for HIV lipodystrophy syndrome [6].

Facial wasting may be severe and distressing for patients who are otherwise stable. The HIV lipoatrophy patient has a characteristic cachectic and emaciated appearance [13]. The face shows progressive loss of orbital, buccal, parotid, and preauricular fat. Eyes appear prominent and hollow. Progressive orbital lipoatrophy causes a flattening and lengthening of the lower eyelids, leading to increased scleral show. Cheeks appear sunken with loss of the preauricular and buccal fat pads. As severity progresses, skeletal and muscle visibility become prominent features. Often, the nasolabial folds flatten and, along with atrophy of the cheeks, gives a prominence to the perioral region. The face develops a simian appearance. For many, this appearance becomes the overt sign of HIV and the source of social, emotional, and physical debilitation [14]. FDA approval of Sculptra, a volumetric and global filler lasting 18 to 24 months, provides a therapeutic alternative for HIV lipoatrophy patients [15].

The Vega study

The Vega study, an open-label, single-arm pilot study of poly-L-lactic acid (PLLA) for the treatment of HIV lipoatrophy, assessed efficacy, safety, and durability over 96 weeks [16]. Fifty patients who had severe lipoatrophy (determined by ultrasonography to be <2 mm facial fat thickness) were enrolled. The median facial fat thickness was equal to 0 (0.0–2.1 mm) and a median total cutaneous thickness (TCT) was 2.9 mm (range, 2.0–5.5 mm). Injections were performed at day 0 and at weeks 2, 4, and 6. Reconstitution of product included 3 to 4 mL of sterile H_2O injection USP. One milliliter of lidocaine was injected locally for pain control. Patient assessment was performed by clinical examination, ultrasound, and photography at baseline and at weeks 6, 24, 48, 72, and 96.

Four patients received only three sets of injections due to adequate response, 26 received four sets, and 20 received an additional fifth set because facial TCT was less than 8 mm. The primary end point was the proportion of responders, defined as patients who had a TCT greater than 10 mm measured at the nasogenian fold (located below the malar bone, ahead of the masseter), at 24 weeks. Secondary end points were changes in TCT and quality of life.

The proportion of patients who had a TCT of at least 10 mm was 19% at week 6, 41% at week 24 (primary end point), 61% at week 48, 52% at week 72, and 43% at week 96.

The median increases in TCT from baseline were significant at all weeks. Median TCT increases of +5.1 mm at week 6, +6.4 mm at week 24, +7.2 mm at week 48, +7.2 mm at week 72, and +6.8 mm at week 96 were documented.

As cosmetic improvement occurred, a significant increase in quality-of-life scores from baseline was noted.

Further benefits of PLLA injections in HIV lipoatrophy are presented in the Chelsea and Westminster Hospital study [17].

Lipoatrophy

Lipoatrophy is not unique to HIV disease. Other disorders such as diabetes, dermatomyositis, panniculitis, and chronic disease states associated with malnutrition and anorexia nervosa may lead to loss of subcutaneous fat. Focal trauma, superficial surgical dissection planes, aggressive liposuction, steroid injections, and cystic acne with scarring may lead to loss of deep dermal tissue or subcutaneous fat. Other contributing factors include genetics, diet, exercise, and tobacco and alcohol use. Fat loss or redistribution is the primary reason for volume loss in the chronologic aging face [18]. As the face ages, the skin develops an undulating/wavy quality. Areas that were once convex now appear concave, such as the temples, preauricular areas, cheeks, and lateral aspects of the chin. The tear trough/nasojugal folds, nasolabial folds, and marionette lines appear deeper and shadowed. Experience and results with Sculptra for global volumetric restoration in HIV lipoatrophy has opened the door for "off-label" use in cosmetic patients who have volume loss. Sculptra is marketed in Europe as New-Fill and used internationally in over 30 countries, with over 150,000 patients treated for skin wrinkles and folds since 1999. In February 2004, the indication for New-Fill was broadened to include lipoatrophy [19].

The Sculptra concept

Sculptra is a volumizer lasting 18 to 24 months. Sculptra's longevity is based on the slow degradation kinetics of the PLLA microparticles, a result of irregularly shaped microparticles measuring approximately 40 to 63 micrometers and having a high molecular weight of 140,000 d. The implanted PLLA microparticles remain and act as a stimulant for fibroblast production and collagen synthesis [20]. Gogolewski and colleagues demonstrated fibroblast activation and collagen production in the mouse model [20]. Further histologic studies are planned for documentation of the PLLA effect in human skin.

Sculptra is not a line filler. For most patients, Sculptra is best used for global volumetric augmentation of the mid and lower thirds of the face. The injector should approach the lower two thirds of the face as a whole. As a three-dimensional (3-D) filler, Sculptra moves soft tissue in a medial to lateral, superior, and anterior direction. The injector should volumize areas that are concave, blending these depressed atrophic areas into those that are convex. This technique allows the injector to establish a uniform 3-D enhancement with smooth transition between cosmetic units while maintaining facial contour. This re-establishes the so-called "bloom of youth"—a full yet contoured face.

A criterion for a volumetric filler is that it must be placed deeply to exert its effect. Whether implanted at the dermal–subcutaneous junction, within the superficial subcutaneous fat, or just above the periosteum (at the orbital rim, zygomatic arch, or temporal bone), the PLLA microparticles are able to ultimately stimulate production of fibroblasts and collagen. The optimal depth of implantation, however, is the dermal–subcutaneous junction.

The mantra "Treat, Wait, and Assess" guides an injector through a Scuptra series, whereas the triad of depth, volume, and distribution of PLLA remains key for optimal clinical and cosmetic success.

As PLLA microparticles slowly degrade, the stimulus for fibroblast and collagen production dissipates. A patient's appearance (in terms of the filling effect) offered by PLLA would be expected to gradually change over 18 to 24 months. As clinical change occurs, touch-up injections may be required. One would expect less total volume or fewer injection sessions required to regain optimal enhancement.

Injection supplies

- Sterile bacteriostatic H_2O injection USP (increases shelf life to 1 month); nonbacteriostatic (shelf life 72 hours)
- Lidocaine 1% or 2% with or without epinephrine
- 3-mL or 1-mL B-D (Becton-Dickinson and Co., Franklin Lakes, NJ) or Terumo Luer-Lok (Terumo Corp., Tokyo, Japan) syringes
- 25-gauge 1-in or 26-gauge 0.5–in B-D needles
- 18-gauge B-D needles
- Marking pencils (eyebrow or lip liner) and sharpener
- Ice packs
- Alcohol/chlorhexidine prep
- Gauze
- Gloves
- Topical anesthetic

Reconstitution

For reconstitution of a uniform homogeneous hydrogel suspension, add 5 mL sterile water injection (USP) 24 hours before injection. For uniform hydration do not agitate but allow the powder-cake to absorb the sterile H_2O slowly over night. Add 1 mL lidocaine 1% immediately before injection, slowly, dripping through an 18-gauge needle. When added too quickly, lidocaine can precipitate the hydrogel suspension, leading to difficulty with injection (ie, clogging) (Fig. 1). To facilitate withdrawal of PLLA, allow the 18-gauge needle to remain in the vial, allowing equilibration with the atomospheric pressure and easy filling of syringes. Do not introduce air into the vial with extraction of PLLA because this may also cause precipitation.

It is fine to swirl, agitate, or shake hard after hydration overnight. Occasionally, there may be a situation in which overnight mixing did not occur. In such cases, the PLLA may be hydrated and held close to the body (eg, in a pant pocket) to "melt" the particles into suspension.

Variations on reconstitution volumes exist. Injectors who use regional blocks or local anesthesia may prefer hydration with 6 mL sterile bacteriostatic H_2O alone without the addition of lidocaine. Others may prefer 4 mL sterile bacteriostatic water and 2 mL lidocaine 1% or 2% with or without epinephrine. Regardless of the ratio of sterile water to lidocaine, in the author's experience, a total reconstitution volume of 6 mL per vial provides an optimal suspension for ease of injection and efficacious results. A 6-mL dilution may further minimize the

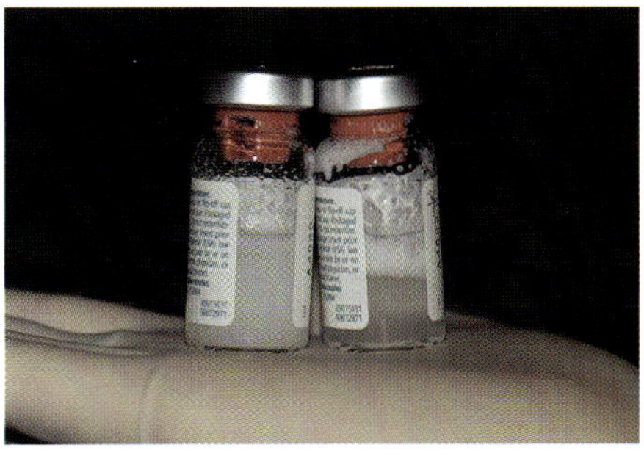

Fig. 1. Add lidocaine slowly to avoid precipitation of PLLA.

possibility of papules or nodules that may occur with more concentrated or less dilute suspensions of the PLLA hydrogel. A 6-mL dilution per vial also provides adequate volume for complete distribution over the lower two thirds of half the face in cases of severe lipoatrophy (ie, one vial [6 mL] per side of the face). Smaller volume dilution, in the author's experience, makes uniform distribution and complete coverage more difficult when dealing with severe cases or larger faces. Those who inject dorsal hands for volumetric rejuvenation have used even greater dilution volumes (10–12 mL total). This higher dilution may decrease the risk for papule or nodule formation in extremely thin skin of the dorsal hands.

Shelf life

Reconstitution with 5 mL sterile bacteriostatic water injection USP and 1 mL preserved lidocaine 1% creates a multidose vial, extending shelf life. One month, stored at room temperature or refrigerated, remains the general consensus on shelf life after reconstitution with sterile bacteriostatic water and preserved lidocaine 1%. If refrigerated, allow to stand at room temperature or to warm to body temperature before injection. This practice aids in suspension of PLLA microparticles. Less precipitation with fewer clogs equates with ease of injection. Date and list reconstitution ingredients and dilution volumes on stored Sculptra vials.

Prep and anesthesia

The patient's face is cleansed with soap and H_2O and the skin is prepped with chlorhexidine (Hibiclens) or alcohol.

Topical anesthetic cream or ointment applied 30 minutes before treatment may help blunt the pain of needle sticks. Ice packs applied before and after injection may mitigate pain, stimulate vasoconstriction, and decrease bruising/hematoma formation.

Given the addition of lidocaine to the suspension, a tumescent anesthetic effect is achieved, minimizing discomfort. Regional infraorbital or mental nerve blocks add volume and may cause swelling, which can lead to confusion with injection volumes of Sculptra and the desired end-point correction. Pain is minimal, given the depth of injection (optimally, the dermal–subcutaneous junction). Intradermal injections of other fillers are more painful secondary to the dermal location of sensory nerve endings for pain.

Pretreatment baseline photos

Documentation of improvement is important for physician and patient satisfaction, especially in a serial procedure that has gradual benefit over several months (Figs. 2–4).

Marking the patient

Marking with an eyebrow or eyeliner pencil, which is easily removed with alcohol, may help the injector plan the case (Fig. 5). The malar fat pad is blended and elevated, thus beginning the restoration of facial volume: elevating concavity and blending to meet convexity. This uniform plane is established while maintaining facial contour. Titration of volume is important as one moves from the superior to the inferior aspect of the face and allows the injector to maintain contour and avoids a heavy or squared off appearance to the lower face. In female patients, this titration restores the more feminine heart-shaped face. Convex areas of skin may be marked with X's to indicate a no filling zone. Facial bone structure also helps guide volume restoration. Planning and individualization of each case is key to cosmetic success.

In the author's experience, it is most comfortable for the physician to inject while he or she is standing and the patient is reclined at approximately 45°. The author usually completes one side of the face and then moves to the opposite side. When treating the full lower two thirds of the face, the author prefers to begin at the most superior medial aspect, the nasojugal fold/tear trough, and to move in a superior-lateral direction to augment the medial, mid, and lateral cheek, followed by the temple and preauricular areas. The author then moves inferior and medial to treat the nasolabial fold and the cutaneous upper lip, followed by the inframalar/buccal fat pad region. Finally, the author moves to the cutaneous lower lip, chin, prejowl, and jawline. The basic principle is to begin superiorly, injecting from medial to lateral, and progress inferiorly, again injecting from medial to lateral. After completion of both halves, one should assess from coronal and frontal views, check for symmetry, and balance the face with a small amount (0.25–0.50 mL) of PLLA that is reserved for touch-ups at the end of the injection session.

Method of injection: retrograde tunneling versus depot

By far, retrograde tunneling is the workhorse type of injection. Enter the skin at a 30° to 45° angle, bevel up. Decreased resistance is felt as the needle passes from the more resistant dermis into the subcutaneous fat. At the dermal–subcutaneous junction, the 25-gauge 1-in needle is easily advanced parallel to the skin surface to the needle hub. To check for proper depth of needle, gently lift the syringe and

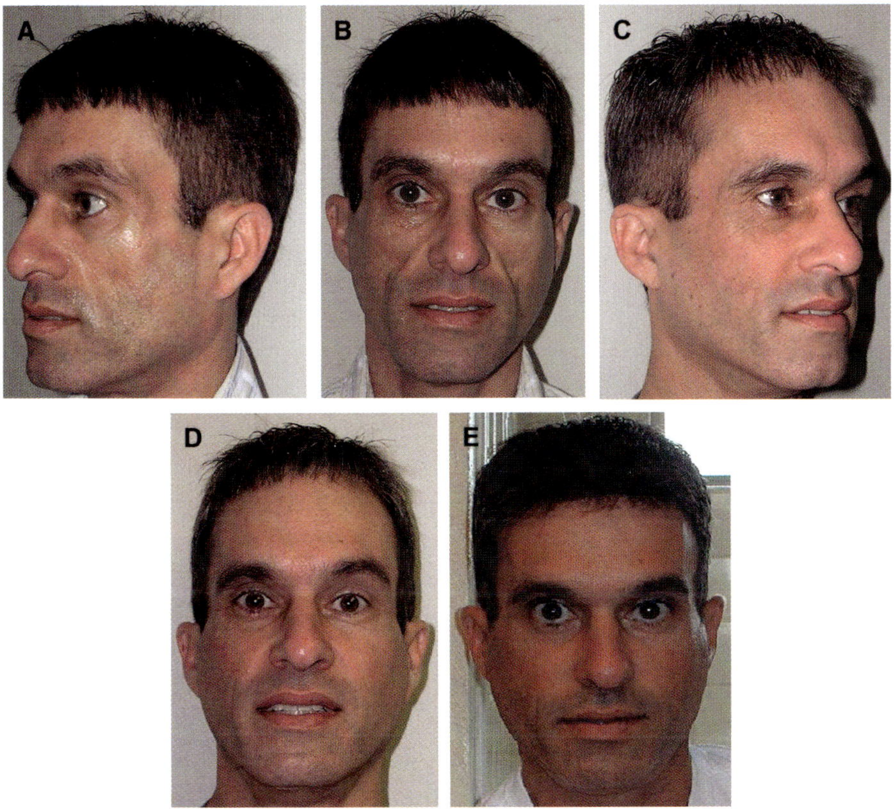

Fig. 2. Case 1. (*A*) 1.14.05, before Sculptra. (*B*) 1.14.05, before Sculptra. (*C*) 07.26.05, after Sculptra. (*D*) 7.26.05, after Sculptra. (*E*) 6.20.06, after Sculptra.

note the roll of skin overlying the needle (Fig. 6). When the needle is too superficial during advancement, the skin will tether or bunch—resistance due to intradermal location. When the needle is too superficial when the syringe is lifted, the skin appears tented over the needle. Withdraw completely and re-enter at the 30° to 45° angle, noting the resistance change, which signifies proper depth.

At proper depth, a retrograde injection is performed. As the needle is withdrawn from the skin, gentle pressure is applied to the plunger and a small volume (0.025–0.1 mL, depending on area) is injected. With initiation of the retrograde movement before injection, an intravascular injection becomes unlikely; however, when the area to be treated is highly vascular, like the temple, aspirate first, begin retrograde movement, and then inject as a precaution to avoid intravascular injection. Tunnel injections are terminated after removal of approximately three fourths of the 1-in needle to avoid superficial epidermal or dermal implantation (Fig. 7). As one approaches the tail end of the injection, less pressure is applied, tapering the trail of PLLA microparticles implanted. It is important to stay at the proper depth to avoid superficial implantation that may lead to a visible papule. Deeper bolus may lead to nodule formation. On average, tunnels are spaced approximately 2 to 4 mm apart. This spacing allows for uniform distribution of PLLA throughout the areas of injection. Again, proper depth, small volumes (0.025–0.1 mL, depending on location), and uniform distribution with cross-hatching in a gridlike pattern ensure safe and efficacious treatment with Sculptra.

After a rhythm is established, these injections are performed quickly and in concert with steps to prevent clogs. Massage frequently post injection. Add ice and pressure when necessary. Some injectors may find it difficult to establish a rhythm of movement. These injectors may tend to "loiter" or "stall" (ie, inject without moving in a retrograde fashion), which is not a good thing for two reasons: (1) without movement, the implantation becomes a bolus injection and may lead to a superficial papule or deep nodule, depending on depth of implantation; and (2) intravascular injection may be more likely. Those who have a tendency to loiter or stall with injection or the newly trained injector should always aspirate before injection.

Tunneling may be modified by creating a fanning pattern in certain areas of the face, such as the temple, preauricular, midcheek, and lateral chin/

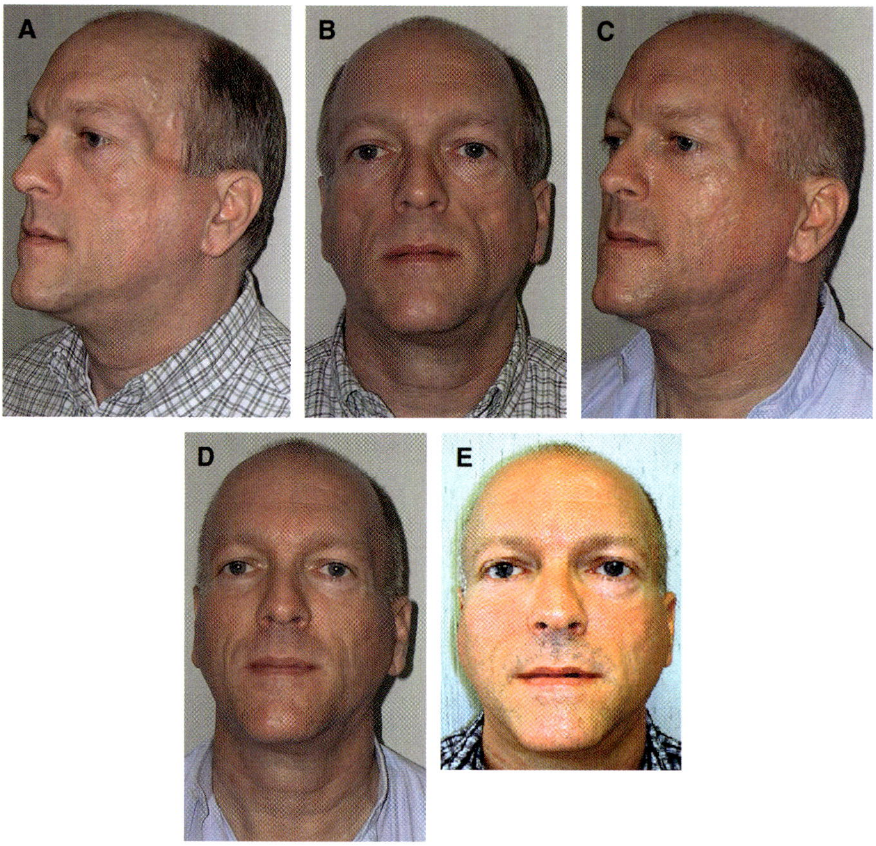

Fig. 3. Case 2. (*A*) 1.21.05, before Sculptra. (*B*) 1.21.05, before Sculptra. (*C*) 6.16.05, after Sculptra. (*D*) 6.16.05, after Sculptra. (*E*) 6.13.06, after Sculptra.

marionette areas. A single entry point and pivotal movement, fanning a series of retrograde tunnels, allows for fewer sticks and efficient placement of PLLA over a broad area. The volume of PLLA injected per tunnel when fanning is approximately 0.05 to 0.1 mL. This volume is injected in a tapering fashion within each arm of the fan to avoid excess accumulation at the point of pivot, avoiding formation of a deep nodule (Fig. 8). Fanning is considered a more advanced injection technique.

Depot injections in the author's practice and training sessions have become less common. Depot injections, by nature, are a small bolus. In areas such as thin periorbital and temporal skin, this type of injection seems counterintuitive and may account for the formation of small superficial papules or deeper nodules. Tunneling can replace the depot method around the periorbital and temporal areas. First, establish depth of injection. For example, in patients who have extremely thin skin, the needle will skirt the inferior aspect of the orbital rim, just above the periosteum. In patients who have thicker skin, the needle may remain within soft tissue at the dermal–subcutaneous junction. Check depth as previously described. At the proper depth, with placement of the needle in the tear trough area, begin the retrograde movement first, then inject from medial to lateral, using approximately 0.025 to 0.05 mL. Icing immediately before and after this injection will stimulate vasoconstriction and minimize bruising. Massage post injection to facilitate uniform distribution of PLLA. Imagine that this small aliquot of Sculptra is implanted over approximately 0.75 in. This technique produces a safer trail or thread of PLLA implanted uniformly over greater distance than a focal depot injection of the same volume.

Injection needles: 25-gauge 5/8-in and 26-gauge 0.5-in versus 25-gauge 1-in versus 25-gauge 1.5-in

Using the retrograde injection technique, shorter needles such as the 25-gauge 5/8-in or 26-gauge 0.5-in require more sticks, more starts and stops, and are more likely to be associated with implantation of a small bleb or bolus of product compared with injection of the same volume of PLLA using

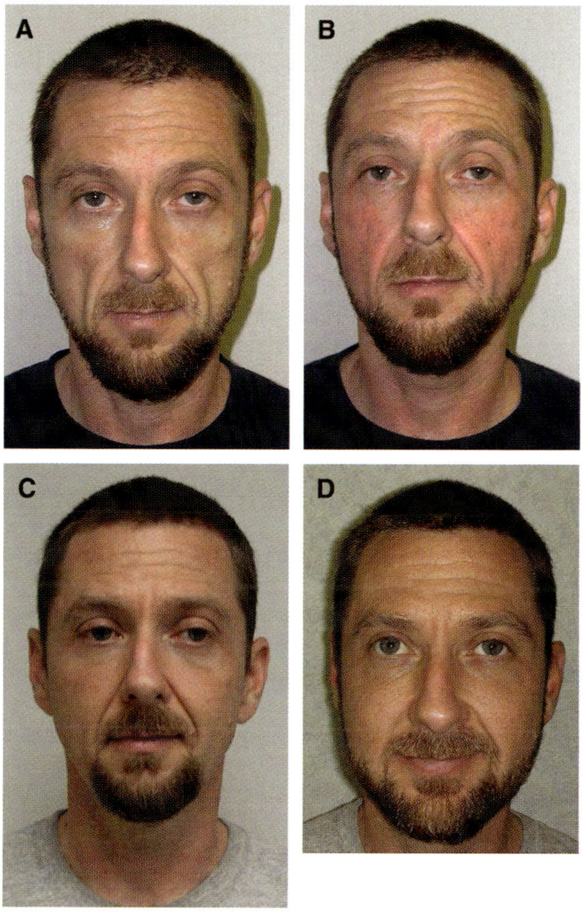

Fig. 4. Case 3. (*A*) 11.10.04, before Sculptra. (*B*) 11.10.04, immediately after Sculptra. (*C*) 7.15.05, after Sculptra. (*D*) 6.06.06, after Sculptra.

a longer, 25-gauge 1-in needle. A small bleb or bolus may be more likely to cause a papule or nodule. The author prefers the 25-gauge 1-in needle, which allows for a uniform tapered trail/tunnel of PLLA microparticles. The 25-gauge 1-in needle may require fewer sticks and is amenable to fanning of PLLA microparticles for ease and efficiency of implantation. A 25-gauge, 1.5-in needle, on the other hand, may be difficult to navigate and to maintain a uniform proper depth of implantation. This longer needle bends easily and is harder to unclog.

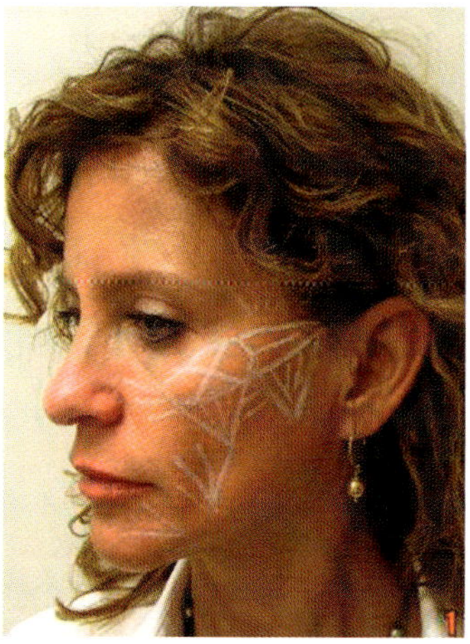

Fig. 5. Marking for PLLA distribution.

Injection: 3-mL versus 1-mL syringes

Agitate the vial before filling syringes to suspend microparticles of PLLA. An 18-gauge needle allows

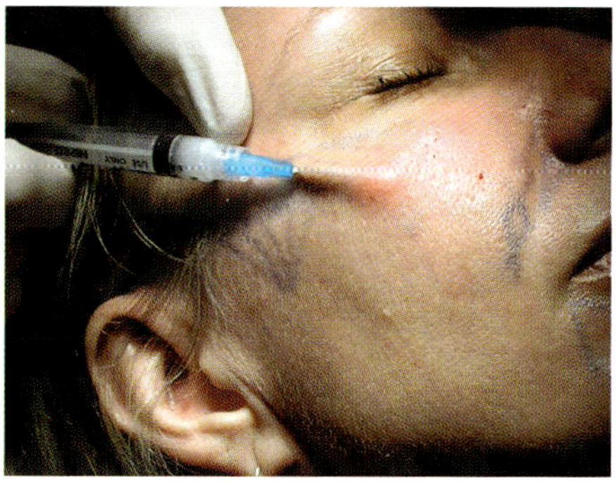

Fig. 6. Photograph shows 25-gauge 1-in needle lifted to illustrate proper depth.

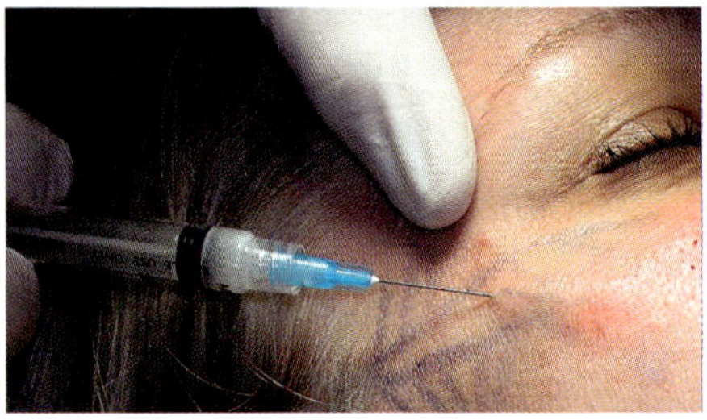

Fig. 7. Terminate injection before removing needle.

easy movement of PLLA hydro-gel suspension into the syringe. Fill 3-mL B-D Luer-Lok syringes to 1-mL volumes. If multiple syringes are filled, leave a small airspace between the hub of the needle and syringe. Resuspend by shaking the syringe and expel air before injection. If PLLA sits in the hub, it will precipitate even before injection. This 3-mL syringe provides a uniform pressure gradient for injection, allowing placement of small aliquots of PLLA with less risk for bolus injection.

A 3-mL syringe filled to 1 mL fits comfortably in the hand. Injection volumes (0.025–0.1 mL per tunnel) may vary depending on area of treatment. After injecting approximately 0.5 mL total, pull back on the plunger, resuspend PLLA micropaticles by agitating the syringe, and express air to avoid precipitation and clogging. A constant minimal drip with the syringe in a horizontal position may help keep the needle patent. The suspension sediments quickly and should be continuously resuspended for ease of injection.

A 1-mL Luer-Lok silicone-coated B-D syringe, on the other hand, may move product too quickly, and the likelihood for bolus injection increases. This syringe filled to 1-mL volume is difficult to handle in smaller hands. If used, the 1-mL syringe filled to 0.5 mL may be more manageable. If clogs occur, resuspension of PLLA may be more difficult given the decreased diameter of the syringe. For newly trained injectors, a 1-mL syringe offers a better visual quantification of small injection volumes (0.025–0.1 mL). With experience, control of small-volume injections becomes second nature, with visual skin movement and correction achieved by implantation serving as the guide.

Injection volumes and guidelines for the lower two thirds of the face

In moderate to severe cases, one vial per one-half face (~6 mL) or two vials total (~12 mL) may be required. Treatment volumes may change based on severity of volume loss, bony architecture, area or areas to be treated, and desired cosmetic result.

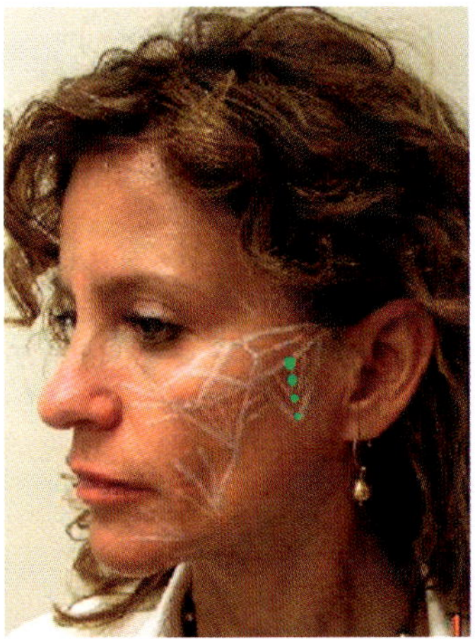

Fig. 8. Titrating volume.

The volumes expressed serve merely as a guideline. As experience with PLLA increases and as injectors become more advanced, the soft tissue response or skin movement following individual small volume injections becomes a visual guide for volume restoration. Massage should be done frequently post injection and patients are instructed to massage several times daily for up to 1 week.

1. Cheeks (nasojugal fold, medial cheek/lateral nasal wall, oribital rim, midcheek, lateral cheek at the zygomatic arch, and preauricular and temple areas): 2.5 to 3 mL per cheek.
2. Inframalar region/buccal fat pad: 1 to 1.5 mL fanned or tunneled over the atrophic area with cross-hatching for uniform distribution.
3. Perioral area (medial aspect of the nasolabial folds and marionette lines, lateral chin, mental crease, and prejowl regions): 2.5 to 3 mL total for moderate cases and 4 to 5 mL for severe cases.
4. Cutaneous upper and lower lip[1]: small trough-like, atrophic area just superior to the vermilion border of the upper lip or just inferior to vermilion border of the lower lip. These areas commonly have superimposed vertical rhytides. **DO NOT** inject the vermilion or body of the lips. Injection into the vermilion border or body of the lips may lead to formation of a papule or nodule. In the author's experience, fillers injected into the vermilion border may sometimes take the path of least resistance—dissecting superiorly into the vertical perioral rhytides of the cutaneous upper lip. This improper distribution and uncontrolled placement of PLLA may also lead to papule or nodule formation. Ice the perioral area before injection. A series of retrograde tunnels, beginning approximately 2 mm superior to the vermillion border of the upper lip, each approximately 2

mm apart, using approximately 0.025 to 0.05 mL per tunnel, is injected. This series of cutaneous upper-lip injections restores volume to the cutaneous portion of the upper lip and will transition into the nasolabial fold. Small volume of injection is accomplished with a quick retrograde movement and by placing gentle pressure on the syringe plunger. Watch the skin closely for a gentle rise in soft tissue. Use a newly filled syringe with homogenous suspension of PLLA, which is less likely to clog and provides a more uniform suspension for refined injections at the cutaneous lip or orbital rim. The steps may be repeated for cutaneous atrophy inferior to the lower-lip vermilion.

5. Orbital rim/eye rings/tear trough[1]: again using small volumes (0.025–0.05 mL), a retrograde tunneling injection is performed at the tear trough area just above the periosteum. In thicker-skinned patients, the depth of injection may remain at the dermal–subcutaneous junction. Ice before and immediately after injection to aid in vasoconstriction and minimize bruising. Often, there is a lateral complement to the medial tear trough that can be filled in a similar fashion at the depth of the orbital rim. The author does not like the depot method of injection in this area. Volume and depth, in the author's opinion, are difficult to control, making superficial or bolus injections more likely with the depot method.
6. Temples: 0.5 mL per temple. This area is highly vascular, so always aspirate before injection. A deep depot injection method just above periosteum at the level of the temporal fascia is commonly used; however, advanced injectors may accomplish uniform volume restoration with the fanning technique at the dermal–subcutaneous junction.
7. Oral commissure: the oral commissure is the only place the author occasionally uses the depot method of injection. Approximately 2 mm inferior and medial to the oral commissure, inject a small depot of 0.025 to 0.05 mL.

[1]Cutaneous upper and lower lip, orbital rim/eye rings/tear trough, and fanning are advanced injection techniques.

Sculptra schedule

In patients who have HIV lipoatrophy, treatments are scheduled at 4- to 6-week intervals for 4 to 6 sessions, depending on the severity of atrophy. One vial per side of the face (6 mL) or two vials total (12 mL) for treatment of the lower two thirds of the face is usually required each session. Because improvement occurs with successive treatments, the volume of Sculptra used may be titrated to lesser amounts or the distribution of Sculptra from one cosmetic unit to the next may be adjusted given clinical response. In most cases, the end point is 100% correction at the time of injection. The exception to this statement may be after the initial treatment of a severe case. In severe lipoatrophy, correction will come gradually with tincture of time if the injector concentrates on uniform distribution of PLLA. Do not overcorrect. Resist the tendency to overfill a severe concavity at any given injection session. Remember the mantra Treat, Wait, and Assess and the clinical guidelines of depth, volume, and distribution of product.

In cosmetic patients, the first and second treatments are separated by 4 to 6 weeks. In the author's experience, total treatment volumes in the first and second treatments are usually matched. Some patients may correct with two treatment sessions. The third treatment may be delayed up to 6 to 8 weeks after the second session, or postponed indefinitely if the patient is pleased with results. If a third treatment is performed, titrate volume as needed but proceed to an end point of 100% correction. Do not overcorrect. Except for severe cases, most cosmetic patients do well with two to three sessions.

The marketing and cost of Sculptra injections allows for further creativity. In the author's experience, patients who require less volume for a focal defect such as a premature familial tear trough appreciate pricing by the milliliter. Others who require far greater volume, such as global volumetric enhancement of the lower two-thirds of the face, may be given a cost per vial. When two vials are used per session, the second vial may be discounted further.

Special considerations

In HIV patients, more atrophic areas are more difficult to inject. With progression of lipoatrophy, the atrophied fat becomes fibrotic. Fat extracted from a patient who has HIV has a cream to khaki color unlike the bright golden-yellow fat from the nonimmunocompromised host. Small aliquots (0.05–0.1 mL), injected in a grid pattern by cross-hatching, facilitate injection of severely atrophic areas and maintain a uniform distribution of PLLA. Examine and treat the patient's face as a whole. Do not treat a concavity as a focal defect. This disease is progressive, and areas of the face may be in different stages of lipoatrophy. Treat areas of mild, moderate, and severe lipoatrophy by titrating volumes of PLLA injected. Blend concave areas into areas that remain convex. In this fashion, the lower two thirds of the face is treated as a whole using the concept of global volumetric filling while maintaining facial contour.

The safety and efficacy of injection correlate with volume, depth, and distribution of PLLA. Small volumes are placed at the dermal–subcutaneous junction, tunneled in a uniform distribution using the retrograde injection technique. With progression through the series of injections, new collagen is deposited in response to PLLA. With neocollagenesis, the increased skin thickness is fibrous, creating greater resistance at subsequent injection sessions.

Expectations

Sculptra series or serial Sculptra injections require that informed consent should express varied results and the necessity of a serial injection technique. If you or the patient is looking for immediate gratification, then this serial global volumetric filler is not for you.

Most patients maintain approximately 20% correction 4 to 6 weeks after the initial treatment session. The appearance does not go down to baseline for most patients. A pretreatment photograph may help keep perspective and expectations realistic.

HIV lipoatrophy shows progressive gradual results with marked improvement in moderate to severe cases occurring after the fourth treatment session. For optimal results, the series is continued for a total of 5 to 6 treatment sessions based on severity and response.

Cosmetic patients may show a quicker response. Most will require 2 to 3 treatments. More severe cases may require a fourth session.

Does Sculptra replace a face-lift?

Sculptra is not meant to replace a plastic surgeon's face-lift. Sculptra, however, may enhance what a surgeon can do with a face-lift. Boxes 1 and 2 summarize treatment guidelines and indications for Sculptra. Postoperative swelling/edema adds volume to the middle third of the face. After 4 to 6 months, the edema dissipates and this pseudovolumization is lost, taking away the healthy, robust appearance of the cheeks. Sculptra may supplement and extend the longevity of a face-lift by restoring volume to the cheeks.

Frequently in patients who have a history of facial surgery, the lateral cheek/preauricular fat pad becomes atrophic, giving the profile a flat and unattractive appearance. Sculptra, as a 3-D filler, can reestablish the lateral anterior and superior movement of the skin, giving the cheek and preauricular areas volume while maintaining contour. Instead of a complication of surgery, this lipoatrophy becomes

Box 1: Guidelines for injection of poly-L-lactic acid

Do's

1. Plan and individualize each case before injecting.
2. Obtain pre- and post-treatment photos.
3. Globally treat and inject the lower two thirds of the face as a whole.
4. Volumize, blending concavity into convexity to restore 3-D appearance.
5. Begin injections superiorly and move in a medial-to-lateral direction, and then progress to the inferior face, again injecting from medial to lateral.
6. Inject using retrograde tunnels and appropriate volumes (0.025–0.1 mL, depending on area)
7. Ice and massage.
8. Follow the mantra Treat, Wait, and Assess to guide through Sculptra series.
9. Think depth, volume, and distribution of PLLA for cosmetic success.

Don'ts

1. Don't fill lines or focal defects with a global volumetric filling agent.
2. Don't loiter or stall with injection.
3. Don't inject superficially.
4. Don't forget to aspirate, especially in highly vascular areas.
5. Don't overcorrect.
6. Don't bolus or inject large volume depot injections (>0.05 mL).

Box 2: Indications: expanding Sculptra use to volumize and refine

Lipoatrophy (hereditary, disease/drug related, aging, and iatrogenic)
In place of cheek implants
Pad aging cheek implants that have eroded dermis/fat
Refine chin implant
Restore cheek volume 4 to 6 months post–face-lift
Volumize the aging post–face-lift patient
In male patients in whom a face-lift is not a good thing
Eye rings or hollow eyes post blephroplasty
Tear trough
Temporal atrophy
Prejowl area
Rebuild/re-establish or refine the jawline
Correct facial asymmetry
Mitigate lower eyelid hyperpigmentation (a vascular effect)
In nonsurgical candidates
No "down time"

a sometimes-expected side effect remedied by Sculptra.

Post-treatment side effects, complications, and care instructions

Most patients have mild erythema post injection due to injection sites, massage, and ice packs that fades spontaneously. Most patients bruise to some extent, which is a likely side effect given the number of needle sticks and injection sites required to volumize the face. Bruising and hematoma formation may be minimized by cessation of common and unnecessary blood thinners such as alcohol, aspirin, nonsteroidal anti-inflammatory drugs, Saint-John's-wort, and vitamin E 1 to 2 weeks before treatment.

Small papules and nodules, although mostly only palpable and not visible, tend to be a source of concern for the patient and the physician. Formation of papules or nodules is most likely technique dependent. Too great a volume injected superficially or failure to terminate the injection before needle withdrawal may lead to a superficial papule. In the author's experience, superficial papules appear to be transient and most undergo spontaneously resolution by way of the phenomenon of transepidermal elimination. In the author's experience, topical retinoids (tretinoin 0.025%–0.1%) and superficial chemical peels (glycolic acid, lactic acid, mandelic acid, or salicylic acid) may also aid in resolution or even help prevent formation of papules. Nodules may also be technique dependent and result from a deeper bolus of product followed by an exaggerated inflammatory response. Nodules may occasionally be visible through thinner skin such as found in the temple or periorbital areas. If the nodule is palpable but not visible and not bothering the patient, then allow it to spontaneously resolve. If it is symptomatic or visible, then subscision with a 30-gauge needle and injection of 0.02 to 0.04 mL of triamcinolone acetonide (Kenalog) 2 mg/mL may be injected to help dissolve a nodule. This treatment may be repeated at 2- to 4-week intervals. Avoid overinjection or concentrated triamcinolone acetonide solutions to lessen steroid side effects (skin atrophy and hypopigmentation). This situation is an example of "less is more." Some experienced injectors advocate subscision followed by injection of 0.9% normal saline injection USP to aid in dissolution of nodules.

If proper retrograde injection technique is used and aspiration is performed before injection of highly vascular areas, then intravascular injection remains unlikely.

Adherence to proper "clean" sterile technique and the use of bacteriostatic sterile H_2O injections (USP) and preserved lidocaine makes infection unlikely.

Post treatment, patients are instructed to ice intermittently for 1 to 2 hours. Swelling and erythema dissipates over 3 to 5 days. Patients are required to massage or kneed the skin several times daily for 1 week to facilitate uniform distribution of product. Sun exposure and vigorous exercise should be avoided until erythema and edema resolve.

Patients on chronic immunosuppressive/anti-inflammatory therapy such as prednisone should be approached cautiously with PLLA. Suppression of the inflammatory response during prednisone therapy may lead to a subtherapeutic response to PLLA. Following discontinuance or interruption of prednisone therapy, an exaggerated or unpredictable response to PLLA may occur.

Summary

Remember the mantra of Sculptra—Treat, Wait, and Assess—and the injection triad of depth, volume, and distribution of PLLA implantation. Be conservatively aggressive; that is, use appropriate volumes at times of treatment, titrating volume to correction, and spacing treatment intervals appropriately. The volume and number of treatment sessions may vary based on age, sex, bone structure or facial anatomy, facial symmetry, cost, and desired cosmetic result. Approach the lower two thirds of the face as whole for optimal effect. Sculptra is best used as a 3-D global volumetric filler, whether or not the patient has HIV.

References

[1] Klein R, Struble K. US Food and Drug Admisinstration. FDA approval of Sculptra for treating HIV facial lipoatrophy. Available at: www.fda.gov//bbs/topics/news/2004/NEW0100.html. Accessed 5/6/06.

[2] Kravcik S. HIV lipodystrophy: a review. HIV Clin Trials 2000;1:37–50.

[3] Mallon PWG, Cooper DA, Carr A. HIV-associated lipodystrophy. HIV Med 2001;2:166–73.

[4] John M, Nolan D, Mallal S. Antiretroviral therapy and the lipodystrophy syndrome. Antivir Ther 2001;6:9–20. [Review].

[5] Nolan D, John M, Mallal S. Antiretroviral therapy and the lipodystrophy syndrome, part 2: concepts in aetiopathogenesis. Antivir Ther 2001;6:145–60. [Review].

[6] Garcia-Viejo MA, Ruiz M, Martinez E. Strategies for treating HIV-related lipodystrophy. Expert Opin invest Drugs 2001;10:1443–56.

[7] Qaqish RB, Fisher E, Rublein J, et al. HIV lipodystrophy syndrome. Pharmacotherapy 2000; 20:13–22.

[8] Torres R, Dadman J, Kassous J, et al. Long term follow-up of patients with HIV receiving rhGH: another dilemma of early versus delayed intervention? Presented at the 13th International AIDS Conference. Durban, South Africa, July, 2000. Abstract WePeB4234.

[9] Chastain MA, Buckley-Chastain J, Coleman WP. HIV lipodystrophy: review of the syndrome and report of a case treated with liposuction. Dermatol Surg 2001;27:497–500.

[10] Carr A, Cooper DA. Adverse effects of antiretroviral therapy. Lancet 2000;356:1423–30.

[11] Berger JR, Pall L, Hall CD, et al. Oxandrolone in AIDS-wasting myopathy. AIDS 1996;10:1657–62.

[12] Gold J, High HA, Li Y, et al. Safety and efficacy of nandrolone decanoate for treatment of wasting in patients with HIV infection. AIDS 1996;10:745–52.

[13] Ritt MJ, Hillebrand-Haverkort ME, Ten Veen JH. Local treatment of facial lipodystrophy in patients receiving HIV protease inhibitor therapy. Acta Chir Plast 2001;43:54–6.

[14] O'Donovan CA, Hourihan M, Petrak J, et al. Psychosocial adjustment to facial lipoatrophy in people with HIV. Presented at the 7th International Workshop on Adverse Drug Reactions and Lipodystrophy in HIV. Dublin, Ireland, November 13–16, 2005. Abstract 34. Antiviral Ther 2005;10:L24.

[15] Sculptra™ (package insert). Berwyn (PA): Dermik Laboratories. August 2004.

[16] Valantin M, Aubron-Olivier C, Ghosn J, et al. Polylactic acid implants (New-Fill®) to correct facial lipoatrophy in HIV infected patients: results of the open-label study VEGA. AIDS 2003;17:2471–7.

[17] Moyle GJ, Lysakova L, Brown S, et al. A randomized open-label study of immediate versus delayed polylactic acid injections for the cosmetic management of facial lipoatrophy in persons with HIV infection. HIV Med 2004;5:82–7.

[18] Donofrio LM. Fat distribution: a morphologic study of the aging face. Dermatol Surg 2000;26:1107–12.

[19] Vleggaar D. Facial enhancement and the European experience with Sculptra™. J Drugs Dermatol 2004;3:542–7.

[20] Gogolewski S, Jovanovic M, Perren SM, et al. Tissue response and in vivo degradation of selected polyhydroxacids: polyactides (PLA), poly (3-hydroxybutyrate) (PHB), and poly (3-hydroxybutyrate-co-3-hydroxyvalerated) (PHB/VA). J Biomed Mater Res 1993;27:1135–48.

CLINICS IN PLASTIC SURGERY

Clin Plastic Surg 33 (2006) 551–565

ArteFill: A Third-Generation Permanent Dermal Filler and Tissue Stimulator

Gottfried Lemperle, MD, PhD[a,*], Stefania de Fazio, MD[b], Pierre Nicolau, MD[c]

When injectable collagen (Zyderm and Zyplast) entered the European market in the early 1980s, it soon became apparent that the products lasted much less than the 2 years predicted by the manufacturer. This prediction was based on animal studies in which 0.5 mL collagen injected beneath rat forehead skin persisted for up to 2 years [1]. Earlier studies on the duration of dermis grafts transplanted beneath glabellar frowns and nasolabial folds during facelifts had revealed that even

Dr. Lemperle is a shareholder of Artes Medical, Inc. San Diego, CA. Dr. de Fazio and Dr. Nicolau have nothing to disclose.

[a] Division of Plastic Surgery, University of California, 200 West Arbor Drive, San Diego, CA 92103-8890, USA
[b] Via Posillipo, 66 – V. le Costa, Naples 80123, Italy
[c] 8 rue de Marignan, 75008 Paris, France
* Corresponding author.
E-mail address: glemperle@aol.com (G. Lemperle).

doi:10.1016/j.cps.2006.09.004
plasticsurgery.theclinics.com

autologous fibrous tissue does not remain longer than 6 months when implanted in subcutaneous locations. Therefore, attempts were made to develop a permanent filler by mixing collagen with various nonabsorbable polymeric powders used in plastic surgery. Histologic examination of these synthetic powders clearly showed that the polymethylmethacrylate (PMMA) microspheres contained in commercially available bone cement stimulated the fewest foreign body reactions when injected subdermally in rats [2].

Arteplast, the first-generation product containing PMMA microspheres, was manufactured and clinically tested in Frankfurt, Germany, between 1989 and 1994. It caused an unacceptably high rate of late foreign body granulomas. The cause of this was a high number of small PMMA particles and microspheres that had persisted during the dry sieving phase of purification because of electrostatic interactions. These small particles stimulated phagocytosis by the invading macrophages. The manufacturing change to wet sieving and the introduction of several washings eliminated most of the particles below 20 micrometers (μm).

Beginning in 1994, a second-generation product, Artecoll, was manufactured and distributed by Rofil Medical International B.V. in Breda, The Netherlands [3]. Artecoll reportedly has been used worldwide (except in the United States and Japan) in more than 400,000 patients [4]. Because of the improved manufacturing process of Artecoll compared with Arteplast, the rate of foreign body granulomas observed with Artecoll is significantly lower; it is reported by the manufacturer to be a rate of 1:5000 patients (0.02%) [5].

ArteFill

ArteFill is a newly developed third-generation PMMA product that meets the rigorous Food and Drug Administration (FDA) quality requirements regarding both the bovine collagen component and the PMMA microsphere component. Clinical trials with ArteFill were undertaken in the United States between 1997 and 2001. For the pivotal study, a total of 251 subjects were enrolled, of whom 128 received ArteFill and 123 received control collagen. ArteFill demonstrated both safety and efficacy in the trial. Subjects who received ArteFill showed wrinkle correction that persisted throughout the 6- and 12-month follow-up evaluations after initial treatment. In contrast, subjects who received the collagen control had returned to baseline by the 6-month time point [6]. Based on ArteFill's safety and efficacy profile, the FDA granted an "approvable letter" for ArteFill in January 2004, but mandated that the collagen carrier be produced in a dedicated facility, according to FDA regulations. The FDA also required that the content of small, potentially phagocytizable PMMA microspheres (< 20 μm) must be less than 1% by the number of microspheres. This requirement contrasts with Artecoll, whose content of small particles is less than 1% by volume. The FDA has not yet granted approval of ArteFill, but this is anticipated in late 2006.

Mechanism of action

Contrary to other injectables, ArteFill is not simply a dermal "filler" or "volumateur" [7], but rather, a stimulant or "stimulateur" [7] of the patient's own collagen production and deposition around the PMMA microspheres (Fig. 1). A key advantage of ArteFill is its suspension in collagen, which continues to keep the microspheres separated from each other for weeks after injection to facilitate tissue ingrowth. Most of the biologic filler materials that increase the thickness of the corium in a wrinkle are broken down by enzymes, or phagocytized by macrophages, within 6 months to 1 year [8]. Therefore, a sustained cosmetic effect can be achieved only with nonabsorbable synthetic substances.

ArteFill consists of 80 volume percent of partly denatured bovine collagen and 20 volume percent smooth, round PMMA microspheres of 30 to 50 μm in diameter (see Fig. 1). This size is ideal, large

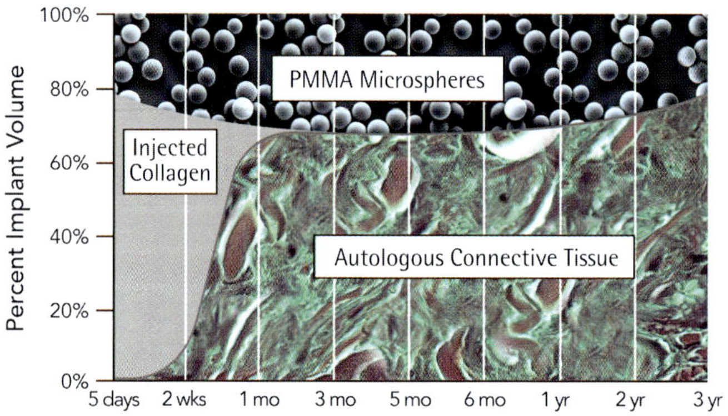

Fig. 1. ArteFill consists of 20% PMMA microspheres and 80% bovine collagen (3.5% plus 0.3% lidocaine). The bovine collagen is replaced by the patient's own connective tissue and the relationship of 20:80 remains constant over the years. Invading microvascularization transforms it into a "living" implant.

enough to escape phagocytosis [9], but small enough to be delivered through a 26-gauge needle. This tiny size also promotes maximum collagen production. The smaller the microspheres, the larger their combined total surface area in a given volume of beads and, therefore, the greater the promotion of collagen deposition. ArteFill's composition allows for a complete replacement of the bovine carrier collagen (80% by volume) with autologous patient collagen within 1 to 3 months of injection. Larger microspheres (eg, 100 μm in diameter) would occupy about 44% of the injection area and only promote about 56% of connective tissue build-up because of the resulting smaller total surface area per volume [10]. One mL of ArteFill contains approximately 6 million microspheres.

Dislocation of the microspheres out of the implant into the surrounding fine network of collagen fibers in the deep dermal layer is prevented by two features of ArteFill. First, the bovine collagen (from the Greek word *colla*, meaning glue) embeds the microspheres and prevents their clumping, thereby allowing tissue ingrowth at an early stage (Fig. 2). This process eventually results in a complete replacement of the injected bovine collagen by granulation tissue (Fig. 3). Furthermore, experience with Artecoll shows that this process continues over the years, converting the injected region into a "living implant" [3,7,8], compared with "inert implants" like collagen, hyaluronic acids, polyacrylamides, and silicone. Second, the 30 to 50 μm size prevents the beads from entering into the interstices between deep dermal fibers, which have a diameter of approximately 10 to 15 μm.

In contrast to the collagen in ArteFill, the carriers used in other injectables, such as gelatin, polyvinylpyrolidone, hyaluronic acids, or methyl-cellulose, have been found to disperse into the surrounding tissue soon after injection. The absorption of these carriers leave the particles or microspheres clumped, with little tissue ingrowth [8], resulting in a harder implant.

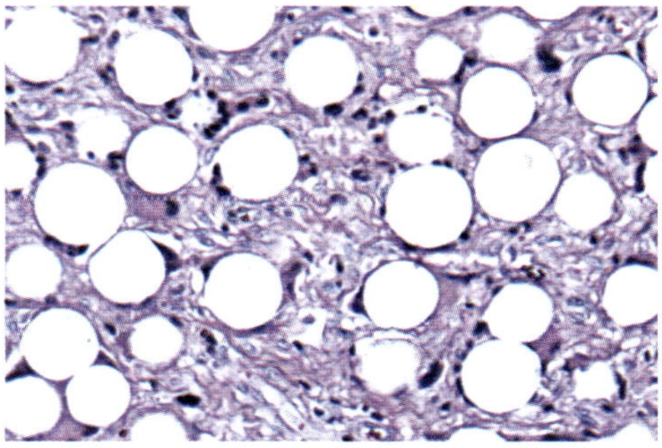

Fig. 2. Histology after 2 months shows the ArteFill microspheres fully surrounded by connective tissue (eg, macrophages, fibroblasts, collagen fibers, and scattered giant cells).

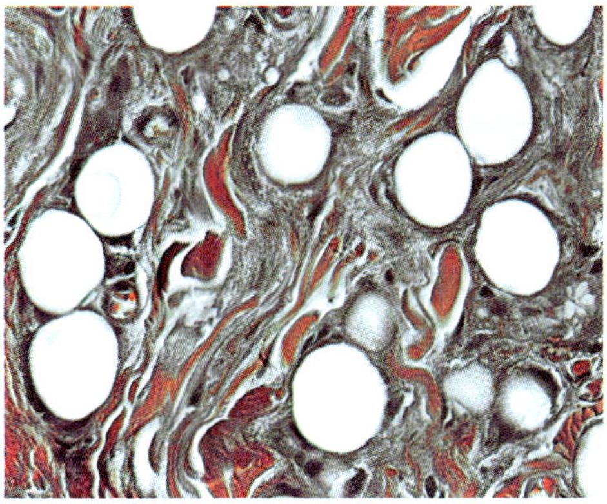

Fig. 3. Histology after 10 years shows a stable implant with collagen fibers still encapsulating the microspheres and making up 80% of the implant's volume.

Implantation of ArteFill produces and maintains a "support structure" beneath the wrinkle (Figs. 4A and 4B) by means of the mechanism described above. Such a structural support prevents further wrinkling and folding, thereby allowing the diminished thickness of the corium to recover (Figs. 5A–5C). This recovery process is consistent with the common observation that, in older patients after facial palsy and in stroke victims, the facial wrinkles and furrows on the paralyzed side diminish over time because of a lack of movement, demonstrating that even in older patients the dermis in a furrow is able to recover its previous thickness. This same mechanism may apply to facial creases after the implantation of permanent fillers, because the creases can no longer be wrinkled to the same extent as before.

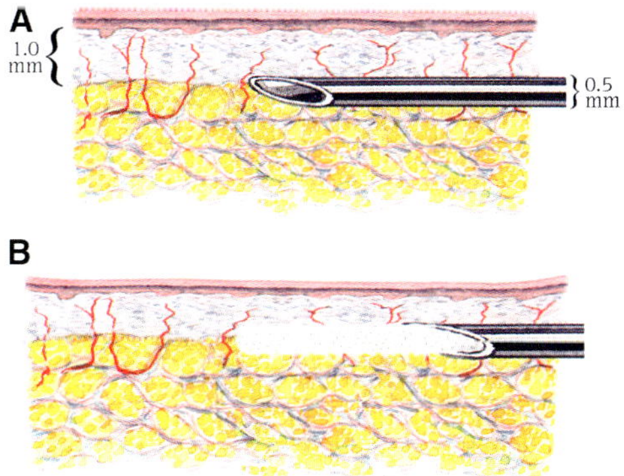

Fig. 4. (*A*) ArteFill has to be delivered through the Tunneling Technique along the junction of the dermis and subdermal fat. (*B*) While pulling back the needle, the tunnel thus created is filled with a strand of ArteFill of 1 to 2 mm in diameter. (Courtesy of Artes Medical Inc., San Diego, CA)

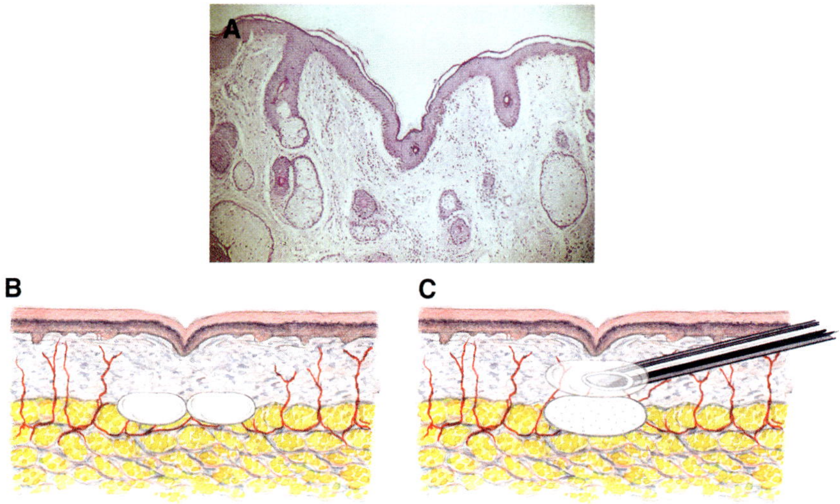

Fig. 5. (*A*) In a wrinkle crease, the dermis is diminished to about one quarter of its former thickness. (*B*) Supporting the wrinkle with an ArteFill "splint" prevents the wrinkle from further folding. (*C*) A touch-up injection causes the thickness of the dermis to recover by itself. (5B and 5C, Courtesy of Artes Medical, Inc., San Diego, CA)

Biocompatibility

Both in vitro and in vivo studies [2,9,10] have documented that the keys to ArteFill's biocompatibility are the extremely smooth surface of the microspheres and the scarcity of particles smaller than 20 µm. The previous, rather high granuloma rate after injections of the first-generation product, Arteplast, probably was caused by the many impurities, such as small PMMA particles, that became attached to microspheres during the sieving process [3]. A correlation between the irregular surfaces of Dermalive particles and granuloma formation has been suggested [5,8]. Indeed, particulate materials, such as polyurethane foam or silicone particles on the surface of textured breast implants, are even designed to cause a chronic granulomatous tissue reaction [7]. Here, the prevalent cells are foreign body giant cells or "frustrated macrophages," which fuse because they cannot phagocytize the polymer or bigger particles.

Histology

Invariably, any injection of particulate materials beneath the skin will elicit a foreign body reaction. As in normal wound healing, the initial event in the response of tissue to a foreign substance like microspheres is the deposit of serum protein at their surfaces.

The second event is the invasion of neutrophils and monocytes, which release their granular components and, in the case of monocytes, rapidly differentiate into macrophages. The macrophages attach to the microspheres and form a one-cell layer on all smooth surfaces. On rough surfaces, in contrast, the macrophages convert into giant cells in an attempt to phagocytize the bigger particles.

The third event is the formation of "granulation tissue," composed of macrophages, fibroblasts, capillaries, and collagen, which fills the interstitial spaces between the microspheres (see Figs. 2 and 3). The bovine collagen maintains the separation between the microspheres, and facilitates tissue ingrowth. Without the collagen gel carrier, the microspheres would clump together, a phenomenon observed with other implant formulations such as Arteplast (bovine gelatin carrier), Dermalive (hyaluronic acid carrier), Sculptra (methyl-cellulose carrier), and Radiesse (methyl-cellulose carrier) [8].

By the end of approximately 4 weeks, the ArteFill implant consists of 20% inert microspheres and 80% granulation tissue (depending on the thickness of the implant). Over time, the connective tissue matures through a natural process similar to wound healing, and the interstices are filled with fibroblasts and autologous collagen fibers.

Histology at 4 weeks shows that all of the microspheres have been encapsulated individually and are surrounded by fibroblasts and collagen fibers. Macrophages are rare and capillary ingrowth is evident (see Fig. 2) [6].

After 10 years, histology reveals strong bands of mature collagen fibers with fully intact capillary vasculature (see Fig. 3). In essence, the injected ArteFill material has become a "living implant." As in normal tissue, there is constant turnover of cells, including macrophages and fibroblasts, which have a lifespan of only a few days or weeks, respectively.

The advantages of ArteFill are as follows:

- **Indications similar to those of Zyplast and Restylane**
- **An aesthetic effect that lasts over many years because PMMA cannot be broken down by enzymes or removed by phagocytosis [2]**
- **Biocompatibility, safety, and stability at the implantation site [3]**
- **Maintenance of volume through permanent stimulation of connective tissue and collagen deposition (collagen remodeling)**
- **Ease of injection despite a viscosity three times higher than that of collagen**
- **No migration potential to distant organs or protrusion through the skin [10]**
- **Minimal foreign body reaction due to the smooth surface of the microspheres [2]**

Allergy testing

Allergy testing of ArteFill is required to minimize the risk of hypersensitivity reactions, especially in patients who are treated with a bovine collagen product for the first time. An intradermal test injection should be administered 4 weeks before the planned ArteFill implantation, although reports of allergies to Artecoll are very rare [11,12]. Questionnaires sent out in 1997 by the former Artecoll producer (Rofil Medical International, B.V., Breda, The Netherlands) to physicians who used Resoplast, which contained the same collagen as Artecoll, revealed only one questionable positive test result among 1280 tested patients (<0.1%) [11].

Injection technique of ArteFill

The method of implanting a particulate permanent filler is more technique-sensitive than injecting collagen or hyaluronic acid. It takes some practice and patience to develop a feel for the correct injection pressure.

ArteFill has to be implanted by the "tunneling technique" or "retrograde linear threading," because its suspension of microspheres in collagen is in the form of a gel (see Figs. 4A and 4B). The advancing needle creates a tunnel, which is then filled with one strand of ArteFill as the needle is withdrawn. One can deposit several strands in a parallel or fan-like fashion to support the wrinkle (see Fig. 5B).

In contrast to the injection of ArteFill, collagen or silicone fluid can be injected through a resting needle, using the "serial puncture" or "microdroplet technique," which results in many little deposits of collagen or silicone dispersing into the surrounding tissue. However, ArteFill remains as a strand within the created tunnel and does not form finger-like projections into the surrounding tissue, as is evident from Artecoll postimplantation histology (Fig. 6). Upon injection, the entire implant is enveloped by a fine fibrin capsule, which prevents any migration or transportation of microspheres into the surrounding tissue. Thereafter, collagen encapsulation of each individual PMMA microsphere occurs within 3 to 4 weeks.

Generally, 26-gauge needles of 5/8-inch length should be used to inject ArteFill. Longer needles offer more resistance to thumb pressure, resulting in lower pressure within the tissue. Furthermore, the thickness of the needle should be used to help determine the thickness of the dermis, much like a depth gauge. For example, the outer diameter of a 26-gauge needle is 0.5 mm, whereas the thickness of facial dermis varies: 0.4 mm in the eyelids, 0.6 mm in the cheeks and nasolabial folds, and 1.0 mm in frown lines (Fig. 7). Thus, the dermis is much thinner than commonly thought; on average, it is only as thick as two needle diameters. This layer is even thinner in a deep crease, where the dermal thickness is approximately one fourth that of normal skin (see Fig. 5A). With age, the thickness of the skin decreases at the extremities, but, surprisingly, it increases in the face [13–16].

As far as implant volume is concerned, overcorrection should be avoided. The deep-dermal tissue layer usually has a certain density that will allow only a certain amount of this relatively viscous filler to be implanted. Therefore, to help optimize results, one or more "touch-up" implantations can be layered on top of the first (Figs. 8A and 8B). These additional injections are recommended at 3- to 6-week intervals because granulation tissue must invade the space between the microspheres. The number of touch-up injections needed depends on the depth of the initial injection and the degree of internal autologous collagen build-up. The latter

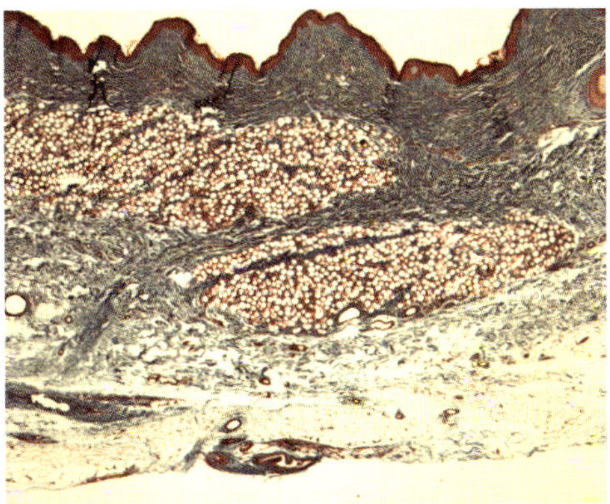

Fig. 6. The microspheres in two injected strands of Arteplast do not spread into the surrounding tissue, but remain as a support structure beneath the wrinkle, causing the dermis to recover its former thickness.

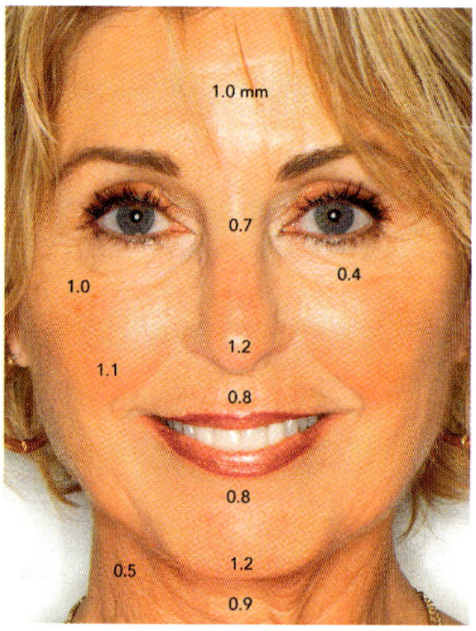

Fig. 7. The dermis in the face has a different thickness at different locations. It varies from 0.4 to 1.2 mm. The outer diameter of a 26-gauge needle is 0.5 mm, just half of the average dermal thickness in the nasolabial fold. (*Data from* Ha RY, Nojima K, Adams WP, Brown SA. Analysis of facial skin thickness: defining the relative thickness index. Plast Reconstr Surg 2005;115:1769–73.)

varies from patient to patient, as has been learned from capsule formation around breast implants. For the treatment of one nasolabial fold of moderate severity, a typical volume of the initial implantation is 0.8 mL of ArteFill. A second treatment may be necessary after 3 to 6 weeks.

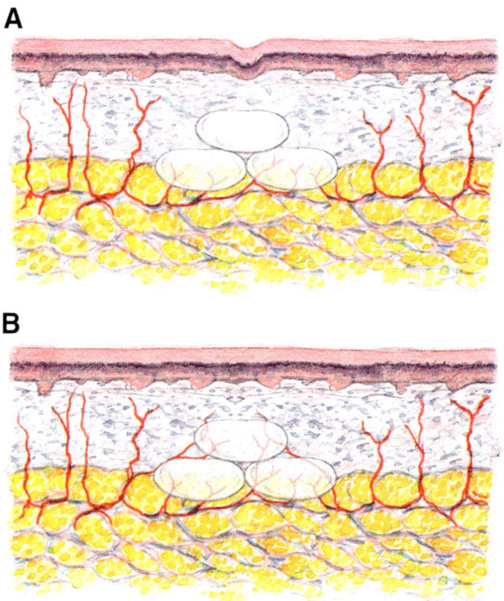

Fig. 8. (*A*) A "touch-up" injection can be administered 3 to 6 weeks after the first injection, when the first strands have settled down at the dermal-subdermal junction. (*B*) The thickness of the dermis recovers and the wrinkle disappears. (Courtesy of Artes Medical, Inc., San Diego, CA)

Injection technique: specific recommendations

Physicians should keep in mind that ArteFill must be injected by linear threading, not serial puncture. The tunneling technique for implanting this particulate filler is described in detail below.

1. Even though ArteFill contains 0.3% lidocaine to alleviate discomfort during and after injection, a local anesthetic [15] is recommended because there is slightly more discomfort during injection, compared with collagen. If there is no indication for a field block, a topical anesthetic (EMLA or Betacaine cream) can be used in very sensitive patients. Typically, it is applied 30 to 60 minutes before the procedure.
2. At the beginning of the procedure, be sure that the needle is not blocked by gently squeezing a tiny droplet out of its tip.
3. Insert the needle with bevel up (while maintaining constant thumb pressure on the syringe) into the skin beneath and along the line of the wrinkle. Begin implanting into the junction between dermis and subcutaneous fat (dermal-subdermal junction), while withdrawing the needle. One can scratch with the needle tip on the dermis from beneath during withdrawing and implanting.
4. Generally, implants are delivered through 26-gauge needles, but a smaller gauge needle can be used in radial lip lines. The best results with all longer-lasting implants are achieved by placing the implant at the dermal-subdermal junction (see Figs. 4B and 5B), not into the subcutaneous fat. The degree of correction in the implanted area varies with patient, treatment site, and plane of implant placement. Correction should be conservative during initial treatment.
5. Resistance from the lower reticular dermis will be felt, indicating the correct plane of placement. If the needle is placed too deep, only slight resistance will be felt from the fatty tissue. If the ArteFill placement is too shallow (ie, within the reticular or even papillary dermis), blanching will be seen. Should the needle be in the papillary dermis, stop injecting immediately and restart implantation one needle diameter (0.5 mm) deeper. The outline and bulk of the needle should be visible through the skin, but not the gray of the needle. Immediately correct superficial deposits by firmly depressing the area with "scraping" motions of the thumbnail.
6. The best cosmetic result can be achieved by depositing 2 to 3 parallel strands beneath each

skin fold being treated, while maintaining constant pressure throughout the implantation procedure. This tunneling technique minimizes possible intravascular injection. The injection pressure is correct if the implant flows slowly and evenly, without great exertion. This technique results in the material being distributed under the fold and outward to about 3 mm into the neighboring tissue.

7. An attempt to achieve complete correction in one treatment session is not recommended. However, overcorrection is difficult when the implant is deposited in the correct plane, at the junction of the reticular dermis and subcutaneous fat. The density of the lower reticular dermis prevents intrusion of the material in robust quantities.
8. Inadequate correction of a defect is usually the result of placing the implant too deeply into the subcutaneous fatty tissue. The defect can be corrected by repeating the procedure with the implant placed just above the subcutaneous tissue at the lower border of the reticular dermis.
9. Immediately after injection, the implant should be palpated by gently applying pressure and evenly massaging with the fingertips to facilitate uniform distribution of ArteFill. Be aware that overly vigorous massage may spread the implant deeper into the fatty tissue, where it does not achieve the desired effect. The goal of the injection is not only to augment the diminished thickness of the dermis, but to support the wrinkle, allowing the thinned dermis to be restored to its former thickness.
10. Patient instructions: The implanted filler can be dislodged from the dermal-subdermal junction into deeper layers through pronounced facial mimicry within the first few days, diminishing the expected result. If ArteFill is implanted inadvertently into muscle tissue, little nodules may form, especially in the lips and corners of the mouth. Patients are advised that there may be some swelling for the first 12 to 24 hours and, rarely, areas of discoloration (bruising) along the injection sites for 2 to 5 days. These are covered easily with makeup.
11. Successive implantations at intervals of 3 to 6 weeks may be necessary to achieve the desired level of correction (see Fig. 8). The second "touch-up" with ArteFill should be placed just above the initial implantation to optimize the result.
12. The physician should instruct the patient to report any evidence of adverse events, as with any dermal filler.

Indications for ArteFill

FDA approval of ArteFill is anticipated in late 2006 for the treatment of nasolabial folds. With respect to unapproved indications in the United States, the Federal Food, Drug, and Cosmetic Act of 1997 allows any legally marketed FDA-approved product to be administered for any condition within a doctor–patient relationship, the so-called "off-label use" of an FDA-approved product.

For each of the following injection sites, a first implantation of up to 0.8 mL of ArteFill will be sufficient: one nasolabial fold, the frontal furrows, both glabellar frowns, both corners of the mouth, or both marionette lines (Box 1). It may be necessary to administer a second treatment after 3 to 6 weeks. In the clinical study, the total mean volume for both nasolabial folds was 1.6 mL of ArteFill (0.8 mL per side) [6]. Cases of patients, who had mandible augmentation or severe acne, have received up to 50 mL of Artecoll over a period of time.

Nasolabial folds

Nasolabial creases are best supported by two to three strands of ArteFill implanted parallel and precisely medial to the fold (Figs. 9A and 9B). During the first few days, the filler still has the consistency of a gel, and may be moved laterally by facial muscle movement. Therefore, it should be implanted directly beneath and 1 to 2 mm medial of the crease. Strands that are injected too deeply are lost and can often be felt intraorally with the tongue. In slim patients, the subnasal triangle often needs

Box 1: **Aesthetic indications for dermal fillers in the face**

Nasolabial folds
Glabellar frown lines
Marionette lines
Radial lip lines
Acne scars
Enhancement of the vermilion border
Enhancement of the philtrum
Facial wasting and cheek depressions
Temporal hollows
Prejowl depression
Single crow's feet
Horizontal forehead lines
Horizontal chin fold
Irregularities of the nose
Bridge of the nose augmentation
Oblique malar depressions
Malar augmentation
Tip and columella augmentation
Preauricular lines
Chin augmentation

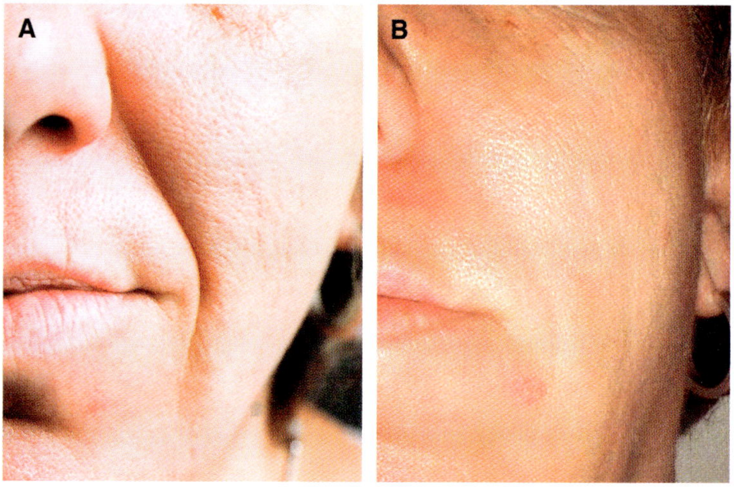

Fig. 9. (*A*) Deep nasolabial folds in a thick sebaceous skin are an ideal indication for ArteFill. (*B*) The same fold 2 years later after 1.2 mL and 0.5 mL Artecoll.

a kind of superficial fanning technique (Figs. 10A and 10B).

On the other hand, care must be taken not to implant too superficially. An excessively superficial implant site may become erythematous for several months, especially in patients who have thin skin, and the implant may be visible in the form of little granules. A second implantation is often necessary, especially in the lower nasolabial crease adjacent to the corners of the mouth.

Glabellar frown lines

Glabellar lines generally pose no problems because the dermis is thick and the connective tissue beneath provides a good support for the implant. To avoid potential skin necrosis and vision loss, one has to be aware of the supratrochlear vein and artery running anterior of the frontalis and corrugator muscles, ie, rather superficially. If a slight overcorrection is necessary, care must be taken not to inject too far caudally; otherwise, a lump produced by gravity may appear. Deep lines and furrows will require repeated treatments. These are the only sites where injections can be placed intradermally, because of the thickness of the skin.

Marionette lines

The vertical elongation of the dystopic corners of the mouth as they extend to the mandibular border can be improved greatly by linear threading and subdermal crisscross implantation of ArteFill (see Fig. 10A). Here, it is especially important to stay closely subdermal because there is no subcutaneous fat between the dermis and the orbicularis oris muscle. In the case of accidental injection into the muscle, the injected strands are transformed into submucosal lumps, which can be felt intraorally with the tongue.

Radial lip lines

Radial upper lip lines extend from tiny notches in the vermilion border and cause the lip to appear

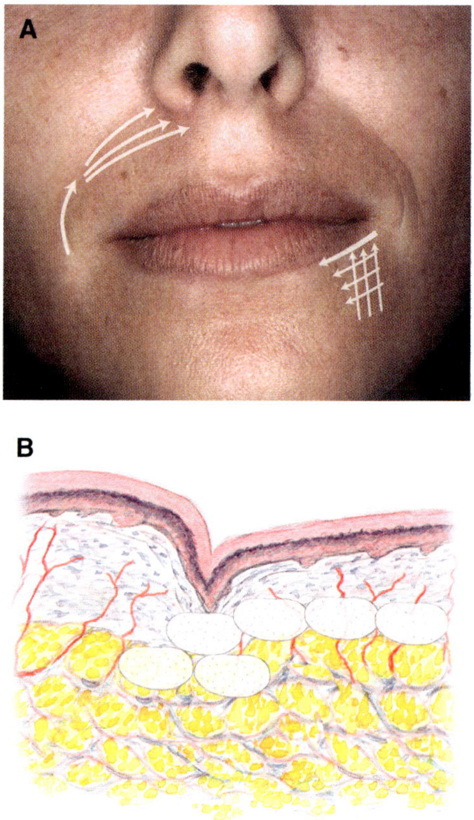

Fig. 10. (*A*) Nasolabial folds often need a superficial fanning technique in the "subnasal triangle," whereas marionette lines often need crisscrossing of ArteFill strands. (*B*) The subdermal strands demonstrate the fanning technique in the subnasal triangle. (10B, Courtesy of Artes Medical, Inc., San Diego, CA)

aged and lipstick to smudge. In a younger patient who has good projection of the white roll, these wrinkles can be treated vertically from above. In patients who have more than four lines, the treatment effect can be enhanced by filling transversely the entire vermilion border (Figs. 11A and 11B).

In the older patient, filling of the white roll and Cupid's bow prevents future development of radial lip lines. Additional augmentation of the lost philtrum from below will give the lip a more youthful look (Figs. 12A and 12B).

Acne scars

ArteFill is effective for mature, mildly depressed "rolling" acne scars and is currently the only permanent treatment option. These scars can be filled either horizontally from a distance of 5 to 10 mm, or, in "boxcar scars," perpendicularly downward directly into the center, while continuously guiding the needle back and forth. Generally, for acne scars, all fillers should be implanted as superficially as possible until the skin blanches. The blanched area can be dispersed and eliminated by pressing the fingernail across it, if it does not disappear spontaneously within 10 minutes. Fresh scars should not be treated because they may not show any improvement and may actually worsen.

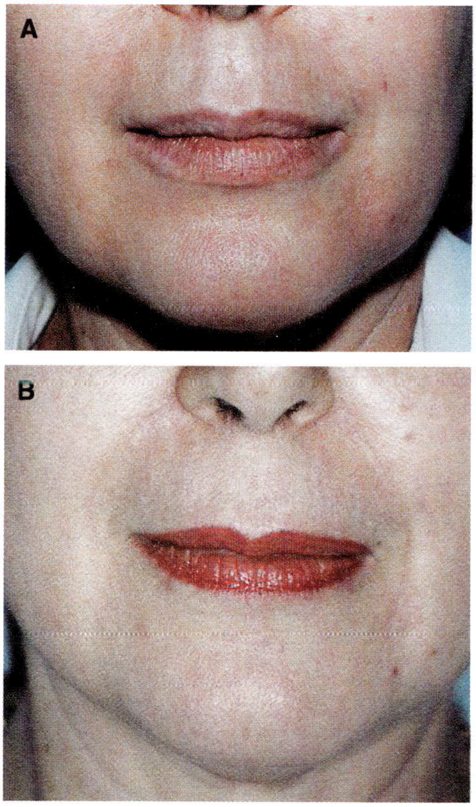

Fig. 11. (*A*) Patient 1 year after removal of Gore-Tex implants from nasolabial folds and lips. (*B*) 10 years after Artecoll in nasolabial folds, vermilion borders, and marionette lines.

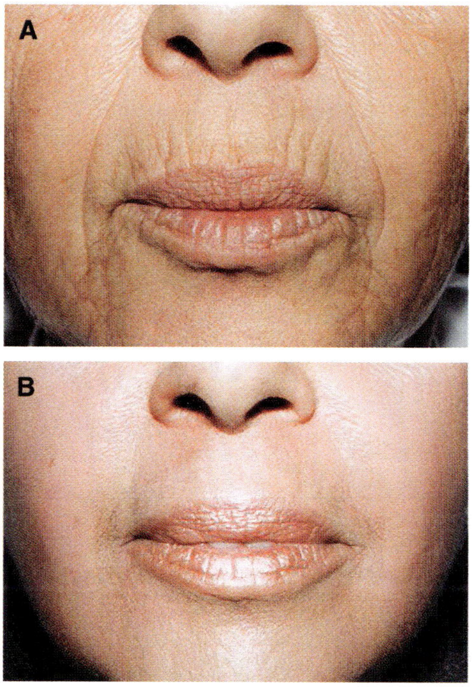

Fig. 12. (*A*) Patient with a total of 5 mL Artecoll in nasolabial folds, radial lip, and marionette lines, and an additional trichloroacetic acid peel thereafter. (*B*) Result 5 years later.

Ice-pick scars require a pretreatment. They should be punched and sutured or subcised with a no.11 blade or a double-beveled Nokor needle at a depth of approximately 1 mm. The fresh wound cavity can be filled easily with ArteFill 3 to 8 days later, after the swelling has subsided and the incision wound has closed firmly.

Facial wasting and cheek depressions

Under highly active antiretroviral therapy (HAART), patients may develop a depression or hollowing of their temporal fossa and their cheeks close to the canine fossa or in the submalar region. This circumscribed atrophy of the malar fat pad and adjacent subcutaneous fat is pronounced in HIV-positive patients who have facial lipodystrophy, which is a well-known side effect of the above HIV therapy. Particulate or some permanent fillers implanted subdermally in mild cases or epiperiosteally in severe cases are of great benefit. In severe cases, the atrophied Bichat's fat pad can be augmented by means of small silicone gel implants or custom-made implants, which may be less expensive than a very large volume of either ArteFill or a semipermanent filler.

Temporal hollows

A common ideal of beauty in China is a rather full moon face. Therefore, many Chinese women desire their hollow temples to be filled and rounded. At least 1.6 mL of ArteFill has to be applied in a fan-like manner on top of the temporal fascia. A more extensive hollow may develop in patients who have HIV and are undergoing HAART; this depression can be treated in the same way as temporal hollows, by applying fan-like ArteFill injections.

Horizontal forehead lines

In deep creases, the dermis is reduced to one quarter of its original thickness. Therefore, the gray of the needle should not show through the skin of the line. Superficial intradermal implantation may result in the formation of small granules, like a fine string of pearls, within the crease. In deeper forehead lines, a second and third session will be required.

Single crow's foot

The only indication for particulate fillers in crow's feet is the case of a single crow's foot in a patient who has thick skin (Fig. 13). In contrast, multiple crow's feet in a patient who has thin and flaccid skin are a contraindication because the implants may be visible through the skin as fine whitish granules. Thin and heavily wrinkled lid skin is better improved by laser resurfacing or botulinum toxin type A (Botox).

Prejowl depression

Prejowl depressions are usually the first signs of a sagging facial skin (Figs. 14A and 14B). If a surgical facelift is not yet indicated, 0.8 mL of ArteFill injected epiperiosteally in the deepest part of the depression will raise the skin and level the margin of the mandible to a more youthful appearance.

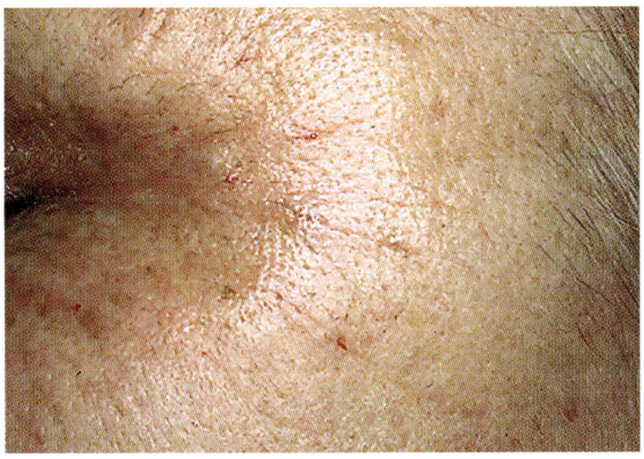

Fig. 13. One or three crow's feet can be injected in patients who have a very thick skin only.

Horizontal chin fold

The skin in the area of the mentolabial fold is relatively tight, and this fold is relatively difficult to fill with any filler. Therefore, most patients will need a second or third implantation. Granule formation in the fold is a danger if ArteFill is implanted too superficially in the skin. In this case, the granules can be removed easily by dermabrasion.

Nose augmentation

East Asians and some Africans with underdeveloped nasal bones often want an elevation to a more Caucasian nose, which may diminish the typical East Asian inner canthal fold at the same time. Through a single puncture in the middle of the nose, a thick strand of ArteFill of about 5 mm in diameter can be delivered from the syringe while scratching with the needle tip along the periosteum from the nasal tip upwards and the glabella downwards. If irregularities or obliqueness should occur during sleep in the first few nights, the patient can still correct the thick strand gently by molding it during the course of about 1 week.

A retruding maxilla (Figs. 15A and 15B), a negative nasolabial angle, or a drooping nasal tip can be raised by epiperiosteal injections of ArteFill under the labiogingival fold.

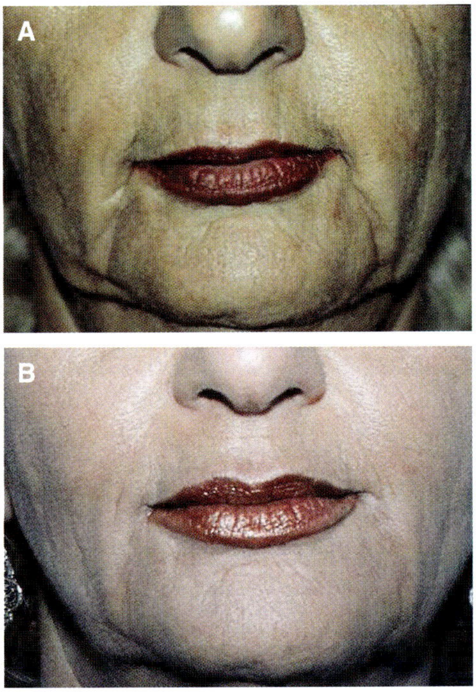

Fig. 14. (*A*) This patient was frightened of surgery but spent her money on 10 mL Artecoll in nasolabial folds, perioral lines, marionette lines, and cheek lines in 1998. (*B*) After an "Artelift" 7 years later, with no intermediate injections.

In bigger defects, a commercially available, harder silicone implant or preformed implant of some other polymer may be more economical than ArteFill.

Irregularities of the nose

Irregularities of the nose (especially after rhinoplasty or nostril collapse) can be improved through deep epiperiosteal placement of ArteFill. The patient should be instructed to mold the implant during the first few days, if necessary. In patients who have an acute nasolabial angle, it may be helpful to implant a triangle of ArteFill subdermally at the columellar and nasal base. In cleft lip patients, the commonly asymmetric shape of the nostrils and the nasal tip can be corrected effectively with ArteFill injections.

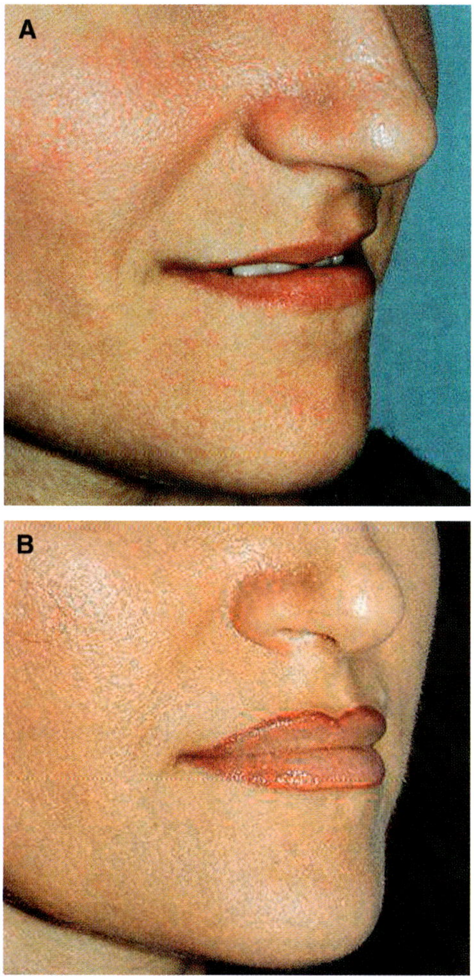

Fig. 15. (*A*) Retruding maxilla and thin upper lip. (*B*) Five years later after lip, maxilla, and chin augmentation with 3.2. mL of Artecoll.

Nipple augmentation

Flat nipples and inverted nipples grades 1 and 2 (eg, those that can be stimulated to protrude) and volume asymmetries can be augmented easily with 0.4 to 0.8 mL of ArteFill. By applying a certain volume of local anesthetic beneath the nipple, the amount of augmentation the patient desires can be estimated. After waiting 10 minutes for the fluid to be absorbed, the nipple is lifted up, and the filler is implanted from above or from the side, moving the needle back and forth to avoid implantation into the ducts. Even if some material does end up in the ducts, it can be removed easily by massage.

Thus far, no evidence suggests that external implantation of even permanent fillers blocks the mammary ducts. The natural swelling during pregnancy will open these ducts anyway. To treat inverted nipples grades 3 and 4, any filler implantation without blind severance of all ducts would increase the crater. Therefore, the ducts should first be cut as deeply as possible, and the filler implanted 3 to 4 days later. Of course, the same procedure can be applied in breast and nipple reconstruction.

Box 2 lists a number of medical indications that have been treated successfully with a permanent dermal filler.

Box 2: Medical indications that have been treated successfully

- Depressed "rolling" acne scars
- Bony defects in the face and hand
- Small skull defects, drill holes
- Depressed temple areas in facial wasting
- Enophthalmos after blowout fracture
- Orbital filling in sunken eye prosthesis
- Tripod fracture of the malar bone
- Flat operated cleft lip, missing philtrum
- Depressed or asymmetric alar of the nose
- Uvula and soft palate stiffening in snoring[a]
- Alveolar ridge augmentation in toothless patients
- Scleroderma, mild Romberg's syndrome
- Facial wasting, facial lipodystrophy
- Visible borders of facial implants
- Shrunken gingival margins
- Vocal cord paralysis
- Inverted nipples
- Small funnel chest
- Gastroesophageal reflux disease (ArteFlux)
- Urinary incontinence (ArteSure)[a]
- Fecal incontinence (ArteSure)
- Intervertebral disc restoration (ArteSeal)[a]

[a] Clinical trials have not been initiated yet for these indications.

Combined treatments

Botulinum toxin

Because temporary paralysis of certain facial muscles does not eliminate furrows or wrinkles permanently, ArteFill can be used as an adjunct to Botox treatment. It can be implanted either concurrently or at a later time. The augmentation effect of permanent fillers may even be enhanced by the paralyzing effect of Botox, which eliminates the motion in a particular wrinkle line and therefore may increase collagen remodeling.

In the perioral area, some investigators have recommended using Botox 1 week before ArteFill because it reduces not the amount, but the power of the lip movement [16]. This combination gives better long-term results and less lumpiness. Six units of Botox are diluted in 0.24 mL of saline in an insulin syringe (0.3 mL, 30-gauge 1/4-inch needle). Then four points are injected on the upper lip and four points on the lower lip, approximately equally spaced. In addition, a few points along the lip are injected at a few millimeters above or below the vermilion border on the upper and lower lip, respectively.

It is important to treat both upper and lower lips at the same time because the orbicularis oris is a first string muscle. Few patients treated with this technique have reported complaints of significant weakness. A similar scheme is also effective in glabellar folds.

Laser treatment

Laser treatment is not a contraindication for ArteFill, but rather a complimentary treatment. Laser peeling of the epidermis can be performed either before or following subdermal implantation of ArteFill. Swelling (edema) of the wrinkle lines and furrows enhances the effectiveness of laser treatment.

The effects of laser rays or laser heat on PMMA microspheres have not been studied. Because "ablative laser surgery" occurs in the superficial layers of the skin and the PMMA is deposited subdermally, lasers in the subcutaneous plane do not produce a temperature high enough to melt PMMA (125°C). Furthermore, the influence of radiofrequency (Thermage) on certain fillers has been studied in pig skin and found irrelevant in this animal model [17]. Theoretically, then, an impairment of the "living" ArteFill implant by laser is unlikely.

Dermabrasion and chemical peelings

Dermabrasion and chemical peelings (Figs. 16A and 16B) are effective in the same superficial plane as laser resurfacing, namely the epidermis and papillary dermis. Therefore, none of these three interfere with the subdermal implantation of ArteFill, which is injected deeper, beneath the reticular dermis. ArteFill can be implanted either before the resurfacing procedure, or months later, when swelling and redness have subsided.

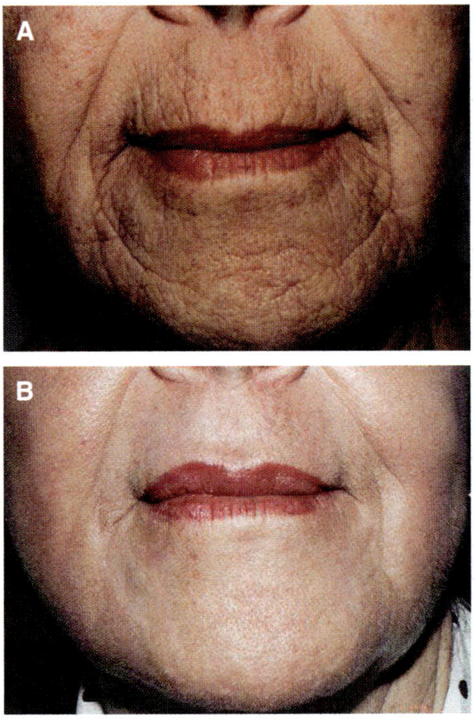

Fig. 16. (*A*) Patient with a total of 6 mL Artecoll in nasolabial folds, radial lip and marionette lines, and a trichloroacetic acid peel (35%) 1 year later and (*B*) 8 years later.

Complications

Technical shortcomings

Because of its long-lasting effect, ArteFill is not as tractable as temporary fillers. Uneven distribution in the form of a string of pearls can be corrected by a second implantation of more filler into the resulting gaps. Most fillers implanted too deeply are ineffective, and the procedure must be repeated. Implantation performed too superficially can cause long-lasting itching and redness, which should be treated with corticosteroid cream or intradermal corticosteroid injections [18,19]. Intradermal granules may be removed by dermabrasion or simple shaving. Excision and suturing is rarely necessary. Dislodged nodules caused by intramuscular implantation should be softened through intralesional corticosteroid injections; however, if they are intraoral, they might require excision. It is important that the excision of nodules always be thorough because any residual filler potentially may cause secondary hypertrophic scarring.

Allergic reactions

Most injectable particles and microspheres are nonallergenic; however, as with all collagen preparations, allergic reactions to these special fillers are possible. The authors have experienced only two acute allergic reactions among more than 3000 patients after implantation of the predecessor Artecoll, and in both cases the patients had negative tests before treatment. Unfortunately, this sensitization cannot be predicted by double testing.

One case of severe anaphylactic shock after eight treatments with Artecoll has been reported [3]. The possibility of sensitization to collagen after multiple injections has been described, and must be kept in mind for other fillers as well. Thus far, neither the histology of excised granulomas nor secondary allergy testing has shown an allergic cause of late granuloma formation with Artecoll. Nevertheless, any late allergy reactions of type IV described for collagen must be considered to be possible following administration of other collagen preparations, such as ArteFill. The treatment of choice is intralesional triamcinolone or prednisolone injections.

Telangiectasia

Telangiectasia may occur at the implantation site in patients who have very thin skin. It usually disappears within 6 months; however, it may require laser or Intense Pulsed Light treatment.

Hypertrophic scarring

Hypertrophic scarring after injectables has been reported and seen in the authors' patients [19]. ArteFill and other fillers are supposed to evoke typical granulation tissue at the beginning and later scar formation in the form of millions of microscopic capsules around the microspheres (see Figs. 2 and 3). As is known from smooth-walled breast implants, this capsule formation can be more or less pronounced in different individuals. After too superficial an implantation of a particulate filler, the treated fold may, in rare cases, develop a hypertrophic scar. However, this scar will react favorably to repeated intralesional triamcinolone or prednisolone injections.

Loss of correction

All short-lasting and semipermanent fillers eventually disappear. In contrast, PMMA cannot be phagocytized by macrophages or giant cells and is resistant to enzymatic degradation. Therefore, the microspheres will remain intact beneath the crease. However, if injected too deeply, ArteFill will remain in the subcutaneous fat, and its effect on the crease will be reduced. This result may occur more often at the beginning of the physician's learning curve.

Additionally, facial muscle movement over several years will push the implant some tenths of a millimeter deeper, and the crease may reappear after 5 to 10 years. In this case, another implant on top of the previous support strand (see Fig. 8) is advisable.

Granuloma formation

Today, true granuloma formation is a rare event, occurring in less than 0.02% of patients treated with Artecoll, with an onset mostly at 6 to 24 months after implantation [5,20,21]. Unfortunately, the pathologist often diagnoses the normal granulation tissue surrounding microspheres as a foreign body granuloma. Histologically, however, a growing granuloma shows a wide distance between the microspheres, and is filled with macrophages, giant cells, fibroblasts, and broad bands of collagen fibers [5].

Intralesional injection of corticosteroid crystals (Kenalog or Depo-Medrol, Diprosone) is the treatment of choice [5,18,19]. The significant improvement of ArteFill over Artecoll, especially the lack of phagocytizable particles, is expected to reduce the incidence of granuloma formation.

Vascular occlusion

As with any injection into the face, ArteFill may be implanted inadvertently into a blood vessel. Theoretically, forceful injection into a dermal arterial branch of the supratrochlear artery could cause retrograde movement of the implant material into retinal arteries, resulting in vascular occlusion. Such complications have been reported with the use of collagen implants and have resulted in the sudden and permanent loss of vision. Similar complications have been associated with other injectable preparations, including fat, corticosteroids, local anesthetics, and angiographic agents [22]. These findings emphasize the importance of avoiding implantation into blood vessels by moving the needle back and forth during implantation and maintaining constant pressure on the plunger.

Treatment of complications

Intralesional injections of corticosteroid for treating nodules and the rare cases of granulomas may become necessary following injection with any implant. Because the granulomas and nodules partly consist of the patient's own connective tissue, the lesion can be diminished significantly by corticosteroid injections directly into the lesion [5].

Hypertrophic scarring, nodules, accidentally dislocated or excessive filler, and real foreign body granulomas react well to intralesional long-term crystalline corticosteroids [5]. Local steroids inhibit fibroblast activity and collagen deposition, macrophage activity and giant cell formation, and swelling, itching, or pain. A 1:1 mixture of triamcinolone (Kenalog, up to 20 mg) and lidocaine, sometimes in combination with 5-fluorouracil [23] or methyl-prednisolone (Depo-Medrol Lidocaine, up to 20 mg), can be injected safely through a 1 mL syringe with Luer-Lok and a 30-gauge needle. Betamethasone (Diprosone, up to 5 mg) consists of larger crystals and should be injected holding the syringe vertically. The injection should be precisely intralesional (ie, into the nodule), while guiding the needle back and forth, because corticosteroids injected into the surrounding tissue may cause temporary skin atrophy.

Because every patient reacts differently to corticosteroids, dose titration is recommended [5]. Two to five treatments at 3-week intervals with increasing dosage may be necessary. Surgical excision can be avoided if this therapy is started early and aggressively.

The risk of cortisone atrophy may be reduced by the injection of an antimitotic agent. For example, 5-fluorouracil (mixed with 1/3 Kenalog or Diprosone and 1/3 lidocaine) [23] and bleomycin have been injected intralesionally into keloids [5]. Minocycline (2 × 100 mg daily) has been given systemically together with prednisone in diffuse silicone granuloma [5]. If skin atrophy does occur, temporary filling with collagen or hyaluronic acids will level the indentation until natural recovery occurs within 3 to 12 months.

Discussion

The aging face loses subcutaneous fat and, one day, autologous fat grafting may become the method of choice for volume replacement [22], as long as its shortcoming of unpredictable survival of fat cells can be resolved [24,25]. Until researchers develop methods to ensure the survival of transplanted fat cells, clinicians must rely on semipermanent and permanent fillers in both healthy patients and those who have HIV-related facial lipoatrophy.

At the moment, hyaluronic acids are the most widely accepted dermal fillers because of their limited persistence and consequently rather short duration of potential adverse events. More and more patients, however, experience "injection and cost fatigue" and ask for longer-lasting dermal fillers.

Among the newer fillers, Sculptra has been of benefit to HIV-infected patients who have facial lipodystrophy because it causes a (so far) unexplainable thickening of the dermis. The polylactic acid microspheres in Sculptra cause a strong foreign body reaction [8]; however, as soon as the body has degraded the polylactic acid microspheres, the effects of Sculptra with regard to volume restoration are also eliminated.

In contrast, Radiesse is very biocompatible, causes little foreign body reaction, and therefore results in very few late foreign body granulomas [5]. Its safety record and reported persistence of up to 1 year make Radiesse an option for those patients seeking a semipermanent filler.

Another semipermanent filler consisting of resorbable hydroxyl-ethyl-methylacrylate particles, Dermalive, which has been used in Europe, Canada, and worldwide, has caused an unacceptable, high rate of granuloma [5].

Injectable silicone fluid is now available with a much higher viscosity (1000 centistoke), compared with 350-centistoke silicone. The newer silicone is marketed under the trade names Silikon 1000 and SilSkin. These fluids, which are 10 times more viscous than water, may not dissipate as quickly into the tissue as the earlier silicone fluid did, and may stimulate much less phagocytosis of droplets by macrophages. The newer formulations are expected to exhibit a significantly lower granuloma rate than their predecessor, which was associated with a rather high late granuloma rate [5]. Consequently, silicone 1000 applied by the microdroplet technique may become an ideal soft tissue filler in patients who have HIV and in lip augmentation.

Other fillers consisting of polyacrylamide gels (Aquamid and Bio-Alcamid) lack long-term results and reliable statistics on adverse events [5,8]. Again, their safety will be determined by the number of polyacrylamide microdroplets phagocytized by the patient's macrophages and by their reaction to a later stimulus, such as a systemic bacterial infection [5].

Summary

The technical and physiologic shortcomings associated with prior generations of PMMA dermal fillers have been reduced significantly since their original market introduction in 1989 [3,5]. For example, the PMMA microspheres in the third-generation product ArteFill meet the new limit set by the FDA of less than 1 particle below 20 μm per 100 microspheres (<1% by the number). Therefore, it is expected that the already low granuloma rate following injections with second-generation product Artecoll (1:5000) will be reduced further with injections of ArteFill. In the authors' experience, which collectively represents thousands of patients treated with Artecoll since 1994, and based on the results in 285 subjects treated by independent United States clinical trial investigators with ArteFill in two clinical trials between 1997 and 2001, both Artecoll and ArteFill have proven to be safe, predictable, and effective dermal fillers [16,26–32]. It is anticipated that ArteFill will receive FDA approval in late 2006 and be marketed internationally.

References

[1] Knapp TR, Kaplan EN, Daniels JR. Injectable collagen for soft tissue augmentation. Plast Reconstr Surg 1977;60:398–405.

[2] Lemperle G, Ott H, Charrier U, et al. PMMA microspheres for intradermal implantation. Part I. Animal Research. Ann Plast Surg 1991;26: 57–63.

[3] Lemperle G, Romano JJ, Busso M. Soft tissue augmentation with Artecoll: 10-year history, indications, technique, and potential side effects. Dermatol Surg 2003;29:573–87.

[4] Artecoll Physician's Brochure 2005. Breda (The Netherlands): Rofil Medical International B.V.; 2005.

[5] Lemperle G, Gauthier-Hazan N, Wolters M, et al. Foreign body granuloma caused by various injectable dermal fillers. Possible causes and treatment options. Submitted to Plast Reconstr Surg 2006.

[6] Cohen SR, Holmes RE. Artecoll: a long-lasting injectable wrinkle filler material: report of a controlled, randomized, multicenter clinical trial of 251 subjects. Plast Reconstr Surg 2004;114: 964–76.

[7] Nicolau PJ. Long lasting and permanent fillers: biomaterial influence over host tissue response. Accepted by Plast Reconstr Surg 2006.

[8] Lemperle G, Morhenn VB, Charrier U. Human histology and persistence of various injectable filler substances for soft tissue augmentation. Aesthetic Plast Surg 2003;27:354–66.

[9] Morhenn VB, Lemperle G, Gallo RL. Phagocytosis of different particulate dermal filler substances by human macrophages and skin cells. Dermatol Surg 2002;28:484–90.

[10] Lemperle G, Morhenn VB, Pestonjamasp V, et al. Migration studies and histology of injectable microspheres of different size in mice. Plast Reconstr Surg 2004;113:1380–90.

[11] Lauro R, Fares J, Brandl L, et al. Post treatment surveillance multicenter study effectivity and satisfaction for wrinkle treatment with Atelocollagen (RMI type Resoplast 3.5% and 6.5%). Breda (The Netherlands): Rofil Medical International B.V.; 1997.

[12] Jellema G. Review report Resoplast user experience. Breda (The Netherlands): Rofil Medical International B.V.; 1997.

[13] Gniadecka M, Jemec GBE. Quantitative evaluation of chronological ageing and photoageing in vivo: studies on skin echogenicity and thickness. Br J Dermatol 1998;139:815–21.

[14] Pellacani G, Seidenari S. Variations in facial skin thickness and echography with site and age. Acta Derm Venereol 1999;79:366–9.

[15] Niamtu J 3rd. Simple technique for lip and nasolabial fold anesthesia for injectable fillers. Dermatol Surg 2005;31:1330–2.

[16] Carruthers A, Carruthers JD. Polymethylmethacrylate microspheres/collagen as a tissue augmenting agent. Dermatol Surg 2005;31:1561–4.

[17] Shumaker RP, Englands LJ, Dover JS, et al. Effect of monopolar radiofrequency treatment over soft-tissue fillers in an animal model: part 2. Lasers Surg Med 2006;38:211–7.

[18] Lemperle G, Duffy DM. Treatment options of dermal filler complications. Aesth Surg J 2006; 26:356–64.

[19] Lemperle G, Rullan PP, Gauthier-Hazan N. Avoiding and treating dermal filler complications. Plast Reconstr Surg 2006;118(Suppl): 92S–107S.

[20] Alcalay J, Alkalay R, Gat A, et al. Late onset granulomatous reaction to Artecoll. Dermatol Surg 2003;29:859–62.

[21] Kim K-J, Lee H-W, Lee M-W, et al. Artecoll granuloma: a rare adverse reaction induced by microimplant in the treatment of neck wrinkles. Dermatol Surg 2004;30:545–7.

[22] Coleman SR. Structural Fat Graft. St. Louis (MO): Quality Medical Publishing, Inc.; 2004.

[23] Asilan A, Daroughem A, Shariati F. New combination of triamcinolone, 5-Fluorouracil, and pulsed dye laser for treatment of keloid and hypertrophic scars. Dermatol Surg 2006;32:907–15.

[24] Lemperle G. What happens to free fat grafts after 20 years in patients who gain weight? Plast Reconstr Surg 2005;116:2035–6.

[25] Guaraldi G, De Fazio D, Orlando G, et al. Facial lipohypertrophy in HIV-infected subjects who underwent autologous fat tissue transplantation. Clin Infect Dis 2005;40:e13–5.

[26] Mok D, Schwarz J. The use of polymethyl-methacrylate (Artecoll) as an adjunct to facial reconstruction. Canad J Plast Surg 2004;12:39–42.

[27] Rullan PP. Soft tissue augmentation using Artecoll: a personal experience. Facial Plast Surg 2004;20:111–6.

[28] Thaler MP, Ubogy ZI. Artecoll: the Arizona experience and lessons learned. Dermatol Surg 2005;31:1566–76.

[29] Broder KW, Cohen SR. ArteFill: a permanent skin filler. Expert Rev Med Devices 2006;3:281–9.

[30] Carruthers J, editor. Review of long-lasting dermal fillers. Aliso Viejo(CA): Medical Insight, Inc.; 2006.

[31] Lemperle G. ArteFill: mechanism of action, injection technique, clinical applications. Submitted to Plast Reconstr Surg 2006.

[32] Cohen SE, Berner CW, Busso M, et al. ArteFill®: 5-year follow-up on patients of the clinical trial. Plast Reconstr Surg 2006;118(Suppl.):64S–76S.

ELSEVIER
SAUNDERS

CLINICS IN
PLASTIC
SURGERY

Clin Plastic Surg 33 (2006) 567–577

Facial Augmentation With Structural Fat Grafting

Sydney R. Coleman, MD

One hundred years ago, surgeons used subcutaneous fillers extensively for altering facial and body proportions [1,2]. This practice continued until the 1920s when complications resulting from injected paraffin and other substances became obvious. Aesthetic surgeons, disillusioned with available fillers, generally abandoned the restoration of fullness as a means of rejuvenation after 1920 and began to focus almost entirely on surgical procedures to remove the signs of aging. Advances in autologous fat grafting in the past 2 decades, as well as safer synthetic fillers, give us a chance to reexamine rejuvenation by restoring the fullness of youth.

Most physicians in the recent past have approached fillers in the face by filling wrinkles, troughs, or holes. But 3-dimensional augmentation of the face for rejuvenation and recontouring is much more complicated than filling a hole. To restructure with fat grafting, the surgeon must not only be proficient in maximizing fat survival after placement, but also must sculpt in a totally free-form fashion from the facial bones to skin.

Development of fat grafting

Fat grafting has been used successfully for soft tissue augmentation since 1893 [3]. In 1896, Silex claimed good cosmetic results in the treatment of periorbital scars with grafted fat. He released skin adherent to bone and grafted small pieces of fat between the bone and skin [4]. In 1908, Eugene Holländer (1867–1932) from Berlin first described a technique for using a needle and syringe to transplant fatty tissue [5]. Four years later, Holländer, who described the first face-lift [6], published photographs of two patients with lipoatrophy of the face, which was corrected with infiltration of fat using his method [5]. Charles Conrad Miller in 1926 described grafting fatty tissue through hollow metal cannulas as a substitute for the subcutaneous injection of paraffin

New York University School of Medicine, 44 Hudson Street, New York, NY 10013, USA
Conflict of Interest Statement: Sydney Coleman receives royalties from Byron Medical.
E-mail address: lipostructure@yahoo.com

doi:10.1016/j.cps.2006.09.002
plasticsurgery.theclinics.com

and Vaseline [1]. He reported that infiltrated fat gave a better long-term correction and a more natural-appearing change in facial and body contours than paraffin. He claimed that using his technique to deposit fat through a cannula gave better results in many situations as compared with implanting fat through large incisions. Even though Conrad Miller reported good results with the injected fat, the technique he described never became popular.

Soon after the early descriptions of suction curettage of fat for body contouring [7,8], Chajchir and Benzaquen [9] described injecting suctioned fat into the face. At about the same time, Teimourian and Illouz [10–12] described their experiences with the injection of semiliquid fat into iatrogenic liposuction deformities. Although some initial impressions of fat grafting were positive [13–16], many of the early pioneers of fat grafting were not enthusiastic about the results with their specific techniques [11,17]. Illouz [11,18] compared the longevity of injecting fat into the face as similar to the longevity of injected collagen. In the late 1980s editorials appeared in the plastic surgery literature by well-respected plastic surgeons denouncing fat grafting though injection based on the early negative results [19,20]. Instead of considering why their technique might not be working, surgeons such as Ellenbogen and Ersek [21,22] publicly denounced the concept of fat grafting as an intrinsically faulty procedure. With more experience, they later changed their technique and obtained positive results [23,24].

Gradually, surgeons have come to realize that transplanted fat can create not only satisfying changes in contour, but also long-lasting results [24–27]. As in every surgical procedure, the success of fat grafting is dependent upon many factors: the techniques and instruments used to harvest, refine, and place fat into the donor site is obviously important, but also important are the volumes of implantation, the sites implanted, the levels of placement, and even the individual patient. In 1926, Dr. Conrad Miller warned, "the end-results in free fat transplantation depend, aside from various local and general factors, on the method and technique" [1]. These words are as much a key to successful fat grafting (as well as every surgical procedure) now as they were 80 years ago. Paying careful attention to technique from 1987 to 1994, I developed the following method for the reliable subcutaneous transplantation of autologous fat, emphasizing respect for handling tissues and basic sound surgical technique.

Structural fat-grafting technique

Harvesting

These steps used to harvest, prepare, and transplant fragile fat tissue have been previously described in exhaustive detail [28–30]. Fat should be harvested as intact tissue parcels that can be inserted through a small cannula but large enough to maintain tissue architecture. Harvesting sites are selected only to enhance body contour, as no clear correlation between donor site location and longevity of the implanted tissue has been demonstrated [31,32]. A No. 11 blade scalpel creates 3- or 4-mm incisions for access. Then a blunt Lamis infiltrator distributes solution into the donor sites. The choice of solution depends on the donor areas and on the projected volume of fat to be removed. For harvesting smaller volumes, local anesthesia using 0.5% lidocaine with 1:200,000 epinephrine is adequate. For larger volumes under local anesthesia with sedation, a solution of 0.25% with 1:400,000 epinephrine is used. Under general or epidural anesthesia, Ringer's lactate with 1:400,000 epinephrine is infiltrated into the donor sites to aid in hemostasis. Approximately 1 mL of solution is infiltrated for every mL of fat to be harvested. Superwet or tumescent techniques should not be used during the harvesting phase since the motion of the harvested fat through large amounts of liquid may break up the parcels of fatty tissues and thereby decrease the potential survival of the subcutaneous tissues.

Fatty tissue is harvested through the same incisions used for infiltration of anesthetic solutions. These incisions are just large enough (usually 2 to 3 mm) to permit insertion of the tip of the harvesting cannula. Fat harvested with this specific technique is with a 10-mL syringe attached to a two-holed Coleman harvesting cannula with a blunt tip (Fig. 1). Larger syringes are more cumbersome and may create damaging negative pressures. During the removal of fatty tissue, care is taken to minimize mechanical trauma to the fragile parcels of fat. A combination of slight negative pressure and a curetting action allows parcels of fatty tissue to move through the cannula, through the Luer-Lok aperture, and into the barrel of the syringe with minimal mechanical damage.

Plunger-locking devices should never be used during harvesting for transplantation. The high vacuums created by these devices or by pulling back too far on the plunger can increase the negative pressure dangerously. This can bring the pressure in the syringe to the point of vaporization, which will obviously damage the fatty parcels of tissue.

Refinement and transfer

After the fat has been harvested, the cannula is removed from the syringe and replaced with a Luer-Lok plug to prevent spillage during centrifugation. After the sealing the syringe, the plunger is removed from the proximal end of the syringe. The syringe is

#1

#2

#3

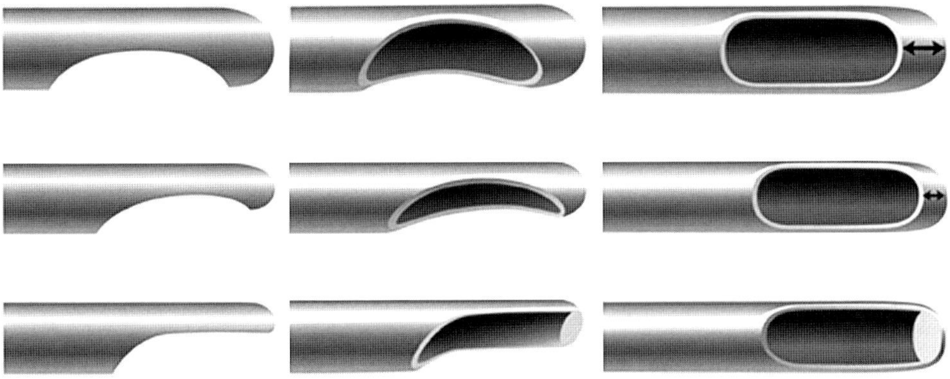

Fig. 1. The Coleman cannula. (*From* Coleman S. Structural fat grafting. St Louis (MO): Quality Medical Pub; 2004; with permission.)

then centrifuged for 3 minutes at 3000 rpm to separate the viable from the nonviable components. The oil layer is decanted and the aqueous component drained. Porous paper or neuropads can then be used to wick off the remaining oil. Care should be taken not to allow the material from the wicks to shred off into the refined tissue. The refined, unwashed fat is then transferred to 1-mL Luer-Lok syringes for use in the face or dorsum of the hands.

Placement

Either general anesthesia or combinations of regional and local anesthesia are the choices for facial anesthesia during placement. The positioning of incisions allows placement from at least two directions into each area grafted. A blunt 18- or 17-gauge cannula with one distal aperture just proximal to the tip is most commonly used for structural fat placement. The shape of the tip, the length of the cannula, and the curvature of the cannula can be altered as needed. Using a blunt Type I Coleman infiltration cannula and a 3-mL syringe, the local anesthesia is infiltrated through the same incisions that will be used for placement of the fat. Vasoconstriction from epinephrine lessens bruising, hematomas, and intravascular embolization of the transplanted fat [33]. Sharp needles are avoided in the subcutaneous planes for injection of local anesthesia or fat.

The blunt infiltration cannula is attached to the 1-mL Luer-Lok syringe filled with the refined tissue. The cannula is inserted through the incisions and advanced through the tissues to the appropriate plane. Unlike the sharp tip of a needle, the blunt cannula tip does not cut a newly defined channel through the recipient tissues but follows more natural tissue planes. As the cannula is withdrawn, fatty tissue is injected into the pathway of the retreating cannula. No fat is placed during advancement of the cannula to avoid placement of the fat in clumps and to encourage nutrition and integration of the grafted tissue by placement in small aliquots. Fundamental to this technique is the placement of fat in tiny aliquots from one tenth of a milliliter to as little as one fiftieth of a milliliter with each pass of the cannula.

Placing the fat in small aliquots maximizes the surface area of contact between the surrounding tissues and the grafted fat. This allows each parcel of fat access to a blood supply and a greater possibility to anchor in a more stable fashion in the new site. Such placement enhances the potential for survival, encourages stability, and minimizes the possibility of visible or palpable irregularities. Dramatic volume corrections are possible by making many passes of the tiny aliquots in one procedure, but this requires time and patience and results in remarkable and prolonged swelling.

Postoperative care

The most expected sequela of fat grafting using this technique is swelling. The many passes of a blunt cannula used for placement of the refined tissue results in remarkable tissue edema. Immediately after the procedure, plastic adhesive tape or Tegaderm (3M, St. Paul, MN) is placed over the infiltrated areas. This remains in place for 3 or 4 days and appears to reduce bruising and swelling. For 72 hours postoperatively, cold should be applied frequently and all infiltrated sites should be elevated.

Light touch can be instrumental in reducing swelling by encouraging lymphatic drainage. However, deep massage of infiltrated areas should be approached with caution in the first weeks after placement. Although it is difficult to move the recently infiltrated fat with gentle manipulation of the area, strong directed pressure could move infiltrated fatty tissue.

Other maneuvers such as holistic medications, low-level laser [34], and electromagnetic therapy [35] may also accelerate the resolution of swelling.

Even with all of these maneuvers to reduce edema, postoperative swelling is still a major factor. Although some physicians report a few days to 2 weeks for recovery from fat grafting [36], my experience is that the recovery can be much longer [37,38].

Complications

A surgeon should be aware of the potential complications be able to avoid them, to minimize untoward effects such as swelling, and to provide an adequate informed consent. The immediate potential complications of structural fat grafting are related to surgery itself. Late complications are primarily aesthetic.

Although the cannulas used are blunt, damage to underlying structures (nerves, blood vessels, muscles, and glands) is possible. The most devastating is the rare complication of intravascular emboli [33]. However, cannulation of a vessel and permanent nerve injury have never been reported using a blunt cannula.

Bacterial contamination of the fatty tissue can result in infection and resorption of the grafted tissue. Meticulous sterile technique must be observed with careful attention to preoperative patient preparation with antiseptic soaps and an antiseptic agent such as povidone iodine.

Fat grafting appears to be stable after placement in most situations. However, during the procedure and in the immediate postoperative period, care should be taken to avoid migrations of the fatty tissue into the surrounding tissues. Forcing too much fatty tissue into any area may cause the fat to move into another area. Placement of fat grafts into areas of significant intrinsic facial muscle motion, such as the lateral corrugators, may precipitate migration from the area of placement. In addition, after transplantation, fat has the potential to increase or decrease in size especially related to weight gain or loss.

Most patients find it desirable to remove fat and contour the rest of the body at the same time as fat grafting. However, a potential complication with this technique is the creation of donor site deformities or problems with incisions. Even the surgeon who is facile at liposuction may create donor site deformities. This is not a complete list of complications, and more exhaustive descriptions of potential complications [38] and untoward effects are available.

Patients

Patient 1

This 42-year-old presented after a face-lift and endoscopic forehead lift (without any eyelid procedures) 2 years previously. After the procedures, she noticed hollowing of her periorbital region (Fig. 2A, C, E). Over a year before, a physician attempted placement of Restylane (Q-Med, Uppsala, Sweden) into her upper and lower eyelids, but the patient noted lumps and a bluish discoloration in the areas of injection.

Fat was placed at one procedure in the following amounts: right temple 4 cc; left temple 5 cc; frontal forehead 4 cc; upper eyelids 1.5 cc each side; right anterior malar fold 1.5 cc; left anterior malar fold 2 cc; right infraorbital rim 2.5 cc; left infraorbital rim 3 cc; lateral eyelid 0.8 cc each side; and each anterior malar region 1.5 cc. Into selected specific wrinkles of the forehead, 2.7 cc was placed using a 22-gauge needle for intradermal placement.

The patient returned at 10 months with subtle, but remarkable changes (Fig. 2B, D, F). She had no topical treatments or change in skin care. The primary change noted was in the quality of her skin with filling of the anterior malar folds (tear trough) and ablation of the wrinkles in her lower eyelids and crows' feet. The pores of the forehead and the anterior malar region were beginning to line up into wrinkles in the before photos, but have become smaller and less linear in the after photos. There is a correction of the hollowing of the upper and lower eyelids, with less upper eyelid showing and an apparent elevation of the eyebrows. The temples area slightly expanded, which allows more visualization of the brow from the front view.

Patient 2

This 48-year-old presented asking for larger lips (Fig. 3A). The following volumes were placed in one procedure: body of the upper lip 2 cc; white roll 1 cc; philtrum 0.75 cc; body of the lower lip 6 cc; marionette grooves 1.8 cc each; nasolabial folds 4 cc on right and 3 cc on left. She returned 2 years after the one procedure (Fig. 3B).

Patient 3

This 22-year-old presented for lip augmentation (Fig. 4A). She had 3.5 cc of fat infiltrated into the body of her upper lip and 5.5 into the body of her lower lip with a blunt cannula. Using a 22-gauge needle, 1 cc was placed into the deep vermillion along the white roll and another 1 cc along the rim of the lower lip. One year after the one procedure the patient returned (Fig. 4B).

Patient 4

This 33-year-old presented complaining of having "no chin and a weak jaw," which he felt made him "look weak and unattractive" (Fig. 5A, B, C). He had a chin implant 8 years earlier and buccal fat

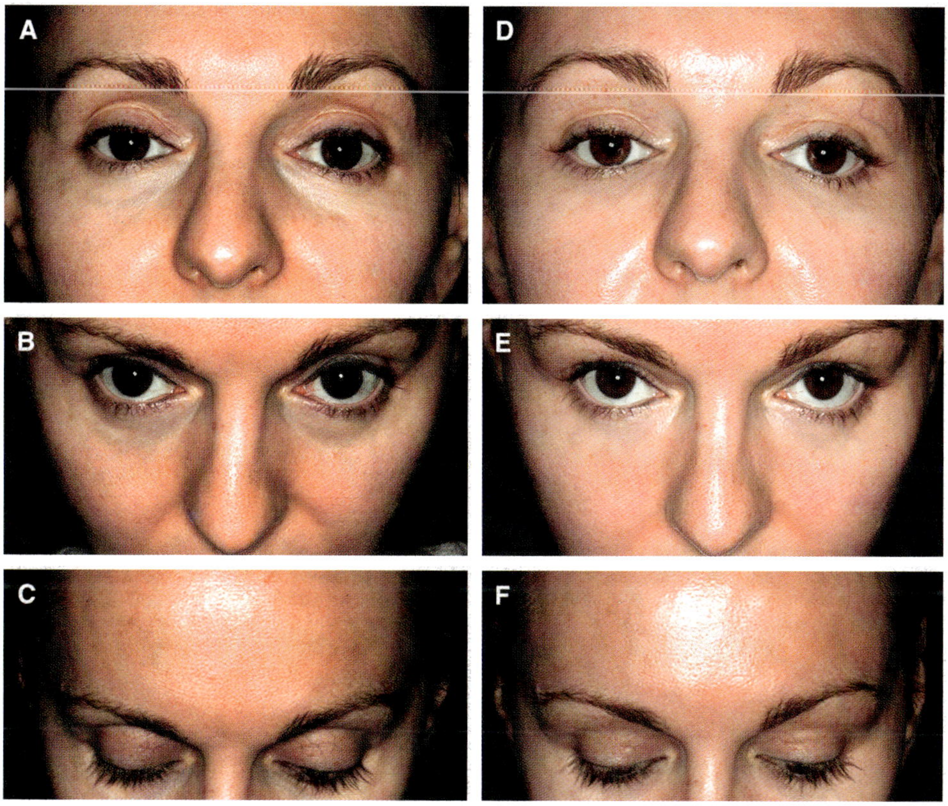

Fig. 2. (*A, B, C*) This 42-year-old presented complaining of hollowing of her eyelids after a face-lift and forehead lift. (*D, E, F*) Ten months after diffuse placement over the temples, upper and lower eyelids, the patient returns with remarkable rejuvenation. The quality of her skin is enhanced with lightening of the lower eyelid skin, ablation of most wrinkles, and a decrease in the size of pores over infiltrated areas. She has a restoration of the fullness of her brow with a youthful decrease in upper eyelid show and an apparent elevation in the position of her eyebrows.

removal 3 years earlier. Along the posterior border, 18 cc of refined fat was placed on the right and 19 cc on the left, both feathering up over the masseter; 8 cc was placed along each anterior border of the mandible feathering up to the lateral chin; and 16 cc was placed over the lower body of the chin. Finally, 6.5 c was suctioned from the right jowl area and 1.5 cc from the left. He returned 1.5 years later pleased with his results, but asking for reduction of the submental region; 11.4 cc was suctioned. He had a more athletic and healthier appearance when he returned 2 years after the submental suctioning and 3.5 years after the only fat grafting to the jawline (Fig. 5D, E, F).

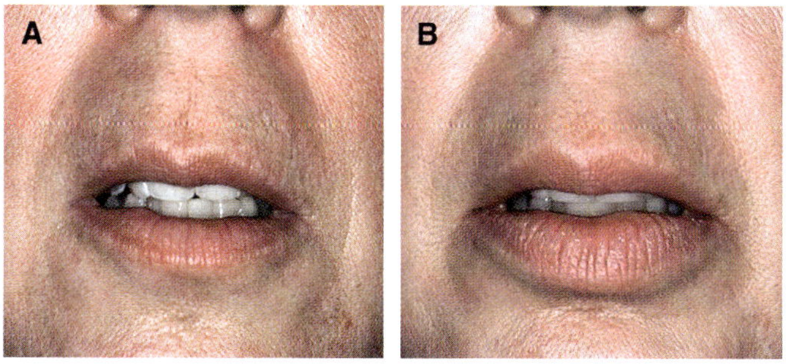

Fig. 3. (*A*) Before and (*B*) two years after one infiltration to the upper and lower lip for rejuvenation and enhancement. Note diminution of wrinkles along the white roll up into the cutaneous lip along with the expansion of the lip to create more vermilion show.

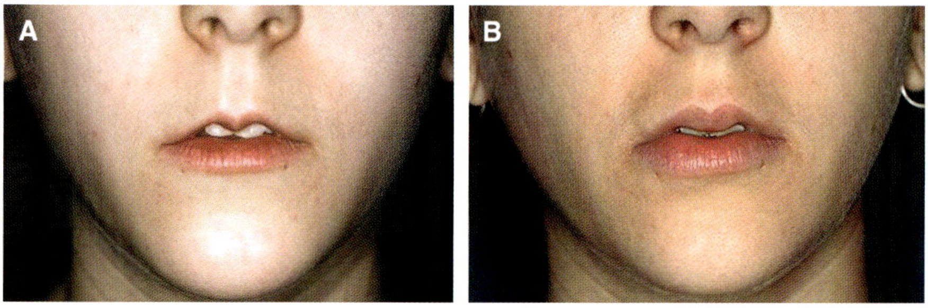

Fig. 4. (*A, B*) This 22-year-old returned 1 year after one procedure to her upper and lower lips. Please note the attempt to maintain the central cleft of the lower lip while attaining central eversion.

Results of facial rejuvenation using fat grafting

These patients illustrate that a full and structured periorbital region, voluptuous lips, and a strong, healthy appearing mandibular border project health and well-being. By using this technique consistently, I have observed that the result from fat grafted by this technique seems to stabilize at about 4 to 5 months. Although a large portion of the structurally grafted fat appears to remain after grafting, research quantifying the percentage of survival with this particular method is needed to demonstrate accurately the percentage of survival.

The goal in facial rejuvenation should include the following: to restore a youthful fullness to the upper face; to sculpt an angular but full cheek that flows into a full lower eyelid; and to create an attractive, straight shadow under the mandible with a well-shaped chin.

Adding support to the midface and lower eyelids rather than excising and suspending structures results in a much more natural rejuvenation and enhancement. The cheek, both malar and buccal areas, is relatively easy area to visualize in 3 dimensions. The results of cheek augmentation with fat are the most what-you-see-is-what-you-get at the end of the procedure of any area in the face and body [39]. I recommend this area for learning 3-dimensional manipulation of the face.

On the other hand, the lower eyelid is one of the most difficult areas for structural fat grafting [39]. Areas of excess fullness and even irregularities or small lumps can be visible through the skin when the swelling resolves. The lower eyelid is not an area to first learn transplanting fat, but should be done when the surgeon has performed enough grafting in other areas to approach the lower eyelid with confidence in the technique.

The upper one third of the face is the least understood area of the face. Although much easier technically to approach than the lower eyelid, the temples and brow require a complete re-thinking of the area to rejuvenate [40,41] (Fig. 2). We have misidentified many of the problems of aging in the upper eyelid, brow, and temple, and excision and suspension procedures do not always work in this area to rejuvenate, and often make the patient look old or sick.

Changing structure of the lips as in Figs. 3 and 4, is a relatively simple procedure, but often poorly understood by surgeons and patients. The process of aging in the lip and the mechanisms for restoring or creating structures in the lip entails not only an intimate knowledge of the subtle curvatures in a youthful, attractive lip, but also the differences between the shape and size of the upper and lower lips [42,43]. A youthful aesthetic upper lip has a distinctly protuberant and continuous full white roll that tapers off from peaks on either side of the Cupid's bow and becomes less obvious laterally. Cephalic to the white roll, the skin curves into a slight concave. The two distinct philtral columns ascend in a similar concave fashion from their origin at the peaks of the Cupid's bow to the columella. Under the Cupid's bow, the vermillion of the lip has a well-centered, distinct tubercle, which is the most caudal element of an attractive upper lip. The width of a lip comes from the most lateral fullness, which is significantly less protuberant than the central tubercle in the vermilion. Between the central tubercle and the lateral fullness is often a concavity or slight depression.

The lower lip has a slightly protuberant rim, which is less distinctive than the white roll of the upper lip. The fullness and depressions of an attractive lower lip complement the upper lip following the shape with opposing components. A distinct central cleft is bordered on either side by oblong protuberances significantly larger than any of the elements of the upper lip. The alignment of the oblong lower lip tubercles is oblique in a fashion that pushes the most central lip out into a distinct pout. The amount of vermilion visible is much greater in a normal, youthful lower lip than in an upper lip.

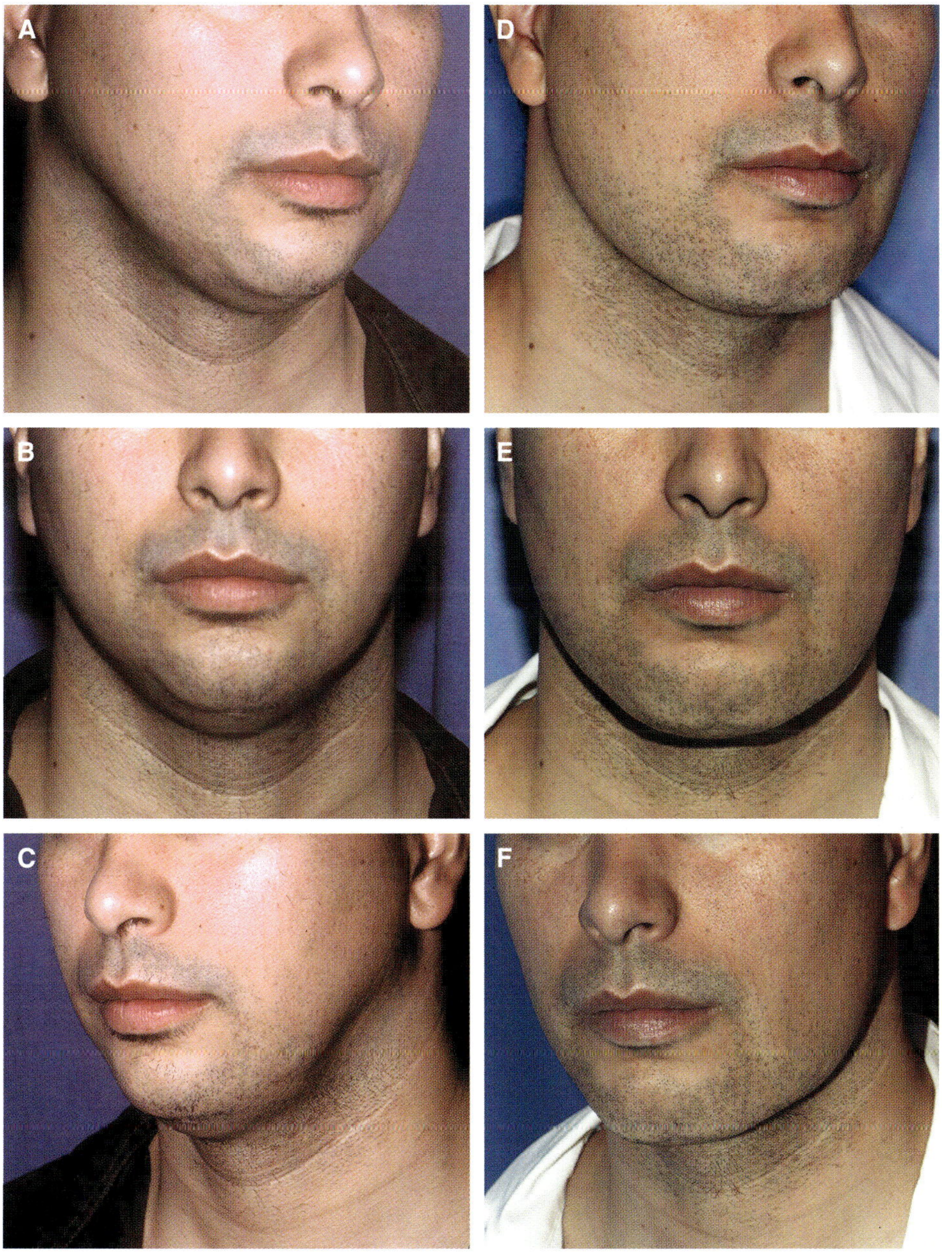

Fig. 5. (*A, B, C*) This 33-year-old presented complaining of having "no chin and a weak jaw." He had a chin implant 8 years earlier and buccal fat removal 3 years earlier. Along the posterior border, 18 cc was placed on the right and 19 cc on the left; 8 cc was placed along the anterior border of the mandible on each side feathering up into the lateral chin; and 16 cc was placed over the lower body of the chin. Finally, 6.5 c was suctioned from the right jowl area and 1.5 from the left. He returned 1.5 years later pleased with his results, but asking for reduction of the submental region; 11.4 cc was suctioned. He had a much more athletic and healthier appearance when he returned 2 years after the submental suctioning and three and a half years after the only fat grafting to the jawline (*D, E, F*).

The lip is not a trough or hole that the surgeon can just fill; instead, he or she must visualize a 3-dimensional structure and sculpt in free form. To attain consistent results with lip enhancement, a well-thought-out strategy that aims at a specific shape for the lip should be devised for every patient. However, the lips are not clay to be molded; they are living flesh with many variables that are difficult to predict: swelling, bleeding, scarring, and so forth.

Strengthening a weak mandibular border as in Fig. 5 creates not only a healthier appearance, but also a stronger more youthful presence. Placement needs to be at many levels from the periosteum to the skin [44].

Discussion

Fat harvested, refined, and placed in the fashion described here has many qualities that make it appropriate to consider by surgeons as the best choice for a soft tissue filler. It is biocompatible, natural, and stable.

The most important concern a surgeon should have of a soft tissue filler is that it should not endanger the health of the patient into whom it is placed. A patient's own fatty tissue, which has not been contaminated by the addition of other substances or microbes, should be nontoxic to the patient and local tissues. Fat appears also to be relatively resistant to infection after implantation, like any living tissue.

Fat infiltrated in the fashion described here can be nondetectable as a separate entity after placement and blend completely naturally into the host tissues. This is because fat has the potential to become completely integrated as living tissue after injection. Although a volume correction from structural fat augmentation is usually obvious on photographic comparison, the changes in structural fat grafts appear and feel natural. Many soft tissue implants can only be placed next to bone or deep in muscle, but become obvious as a separate entity with superficial placement. Likewise, some injectable fillers are approved only for dermal injections. Structural fat can be placed superficially and deeply into most levels of the face.

Harvesting and refinement

Fat is fragile tissue that may not survive the trauma of harvesting, refinement, transfer, and insertion into a donor site. Each step has the potential to injure the fat cell or destroy the fatty tissue architecture. The survival of free grafts of most human tissue (skin, bone, cartilage, cornea, and so forth) requires maintenance of tissue architecture, not just the transplantation of cells. The most important consideration for harvesting and refinement in preparation for grafting is to respect and maintain the tissue architecture of living fat. Any mechanical or chemical insult that damages the fragile tissue architecture of fat will result in eventual necrosis of the injected fat.

Fat should be harvested as an intact parcel already a size that can easily pass through the lumen of the small infiltration cannula to allow placement. The mechanical activities used to reduce large parcel sizes to allow passage through a smaller needle (straining, chopping, beating, washing) potentially fatally disrupt the fragile tissue architecture. For predictable results, the surgeon should refine the fat into relatively pure living tissue. Transplanting a high percentage of nonviable components (oil, blood, local) reduces the potential for accurate volume estimation.

Placement

The transplanted fat must have access to a blood supply. This technique emphasizes integrated placement of fat with fat parcel separated from each other and the host tissue in between. This places each parcel in maximal contact with vascularized host tissues rather than other pieces of fat. It also encourages anchoring of the fat parcels to the host tissue, which discourages migration in the immediate postoperative period. Placement in this manner allows integration of the transplanted tissue into the host tissue so that the fat is not palpable as a discrete entity.

Using this technique, the fat should be grafted so that the desired shapes are formed during the infiltration of the fat. Because the fat is integrated into the host tissue using this technique, attempts at significant molding of the fat after placement are usually futile and can cause undesirable irregularities.

Volumes of placement

The key to accurate volume placement is familiarity with the technique, knowledge of attractive facial topography, and understanding the goals of the patient. A surgeon must understand facial proportion and the manner that fullness is lost with age.

With experience, the surgeon comes to expect what 5 mL of refined fat will do when placed in the cheek, lower eyelid, lip, or chin. However, even with a preconceived idea of the amount to place in any area, the shape and size of the area immediately after grafting is an important clue for determining the volume and placement of fat.

Unfortunately, many variables can alter the appearance immediately after grafting. The edema caused by forcing a blunt cannula repeatedly through the tissue can be different from person to person as well as area to area. A hematoma or even excessive bruising can mislead the surgeon. In areas of strong facial muscle movement (mouth, glabela), motion may play a role in some patients in forcing the infiltrated fat out of the area of placement in the immediate postoperative period. Not only are there many local factors that influence the ability of fat grafts to enact certain corrections by a volume placed, but also there are genetic, dietary, pharmaceutical, and other factors yet to be determined.

Levels for placement

Surgeons sculpting the face with autologous fat must address the many different levels, anatomical compartments, and structures such as bone, muscle, fascia, major salivary glands, nerves, blood vessels, and skin. I have described in the past placement of fat at all levels from the periosteum, perichondrium, or mucosa to the subdermis or vermilion. However, I now avoid placement of fat into facial muscles in most situations as it creates superficial edema, which deceives a surgeon into believing that a correction has been attained. For instance, placement of fat into the obicularis oris will create submucosal and subvermillion swelling that will evert the lip. However, as the superficial swelling subsides from under the mucosa and vermillion, the lip inverts. This leaves a thicker muscle in the lip without the correction afforded by the eversion of the vermillion and mucosa. Therefore, in a front photograph, the lip will not appear to have increased in size because it is no longer everted even though the fat has survived. Instead, in a profile view the lips will project away from the face in an unnatural fashion.

Intradermal placement

I have specifically discouraged intradermal placement in the past [45]; however, in the past 3 years as I began to use hyaluronic acid in my practice, I became reacquainted with the advantages of intradermal augmentation. With that in mind, for scars and deep wrinkles, I now use a sharp 22-gauge needle to place small amounts of fat into the deep dermis to complement the subcutaneous placement. Forcing large parcels of fat through a needle is technically awkward, and the needles block frequently. Particular care should be paid to avoiding placement that is isolated since such corrections may result in circumscribed, visible corrections. The long-term effect of this method of placement does not appear to be as reliable as with subcutaneous placement with a larger bore cannula. However, I have observed significant correction for 2 years in some patients; furthermore, the effect of intradermal placement of fat is different from the effect of placement of the same volume into deeper subcutaneous planes. With intradermal placement, wrinkles can be softened or even ablated with minimal volume. Scars can be improved or eliminated that would not be as affected by simple subcutaneous placement.

Release of adhesions

This intradermal technique of fat placement is specifically different from the technique of injection with a sharp needle into a subcutaneous plane described by Carraway and Mellow [13]. They described the use of small sharp needles to undermine before placement with the needle. This may create a potential space that can destabilize the placement of fat and encourage migration and irregularities. Therefore, I do not recommend undermining before injection. If adhesions, scars, or ligaments are still present after the initial placement of fat subcutaneously and intradermally, it may be necessary to release them with a "v-dissector" or sharp needle in a "subcision" fashion [46]. In these instances, the sharp instrument is used to disrupt a connection from the dermis to the underlying anatomic structures. This type of maneuver is traumatic and may allow the placed fat to migrate. Such destabilizing approaches should be used with caution and should be delayed until after intradermal and subcutaneous placement is substantially completed.

Research

Fat grafting is technique dependent, and not all techniques, surgeons, and patients will experience the same longevity or effect of grafted fat. One of the current problems with analysis of the results of fat grafting is that there has been never been a standardization of the methods of fat grafting used. Radically different techniques are often used in both research and in clinical practices, which makes extrapolation of the result of studies or anecdotal experiences to other situations difficult. In addition, remarkable ranges of the results have been noted from one human to another and between different anatomical sites even when using exactly the same technique and volumes [47]. Surgeons should try to identify the techniques, patients, and anatomic regions that encourage long-term survival and reliable results with grafted fatty tissue.

Summary

The outcome of grafting fat is dependent upon variations in the technique used to harvest, refine, transfer, and place fat as well as the avoidance of complications. In addition, the effects of grafted fat differ between recipient sites and even from patient to patient. Because of this variability and perhaps because of other factors not understood, the results of fat grafting with some techniques, in some patients, and in some areas can be unpredictable. Directed research will help us to understand better the differences between different techniques, surgeons, and patients for this valuable technique and to elucidate the methods and situations that will provide surgeons with the most consistent results.

Fat grafting through a blunt cannula has been used by plastic surgeons for altering facial contours for almost 100 years. Autologous tissue is completely biocompatible, and therefore is usually the safest choice for altering facial volume or contours. Furthermore, fat grafts can be placed in such a fashion that they are long lasting, completely integrated, and natural appearing. However, only in the past 20 years have advances in techniques and instrumentation allowed us to obtain predictable results that make fat grafting a viable option for soft tissue augmentation. Concurrent with the development of fat grafting, our understanding of aging and methods of rejuvenation have developed also. We now approach rejuvenation and adjustment of facial proportion with a better understanding of the need for the restoration or adjustment of facial volume.

References

[1] Miller JJ, Popp JC. Fat hypertrophy after autologous fat transfer. Ophthal Plast Reconstr Surg 2002;18(3):228–31.

[2] Kolle FS. Plastic and cosmetic surgery. New York: Appleton; 1911.

[3] Neuber F. Fettransplantation. Bericht über die Verhandlungen der Deutschen Gesellschaft für Chirurgie. Zentralbl Chir 1893;22:66 [in German].

[4] Neuhof H, Hirshfeld S. The transplantation of tissues. New York: D. Appleton and Company; 1923.

[5] Holländer E. Plastik und Medizin. Stuttgart: Ferdinand Enke; 1912.

[6] Rogers BO. The development of aesthetic plastic surgery: a history. Aesthetic Plast Surg 1976;1(1):3–24.

[7] Kesselring UK, Meyer R. A suction curette for removal of excessive local deposits of subcutaneous fat. Plast Reconstr Surg 1978;62(2):305–6.

[8] Teimourian B, Fisher JB. Suction curettage to remove excess fat for body contouring. Plast Reconstr Surg 1981;68(1):50–8.

[9] Chajchir A, Benzaquen I. Liposuction fat grafts in face wrinkles and hemifacial atrophy. Aesthetic Plast Surg 1986;10(2):115–7.

[10] Teimourian B. Repair of soft-tissue contour deficit by means of semiliquid fat graft. Plast Reconstr Surg 1986;78(1):123–4.

[11] Illouz YG. The fat cell "graft": a new technique to fill depressions. Plast Reconstr Surg 1986;78(1):122–3.

[12] Illouz Y-G. Liposuction: the Franco-American experience. Beverly Hills (CA): Medical Aesthetic, Inc.; 1985.

[13] Carraway JH, Mellow CG. Syringe aspiration and fat concentration: a simple technique for autologous fat injection. Ann Plast Surg 1990;24(3):293–6.

[14] Lewis CM. Transplantation of autologous fat. Plast Reconstr Surg 1991;88(6):1110–1.

[15] Fournier PF. Facial recontouring with fat grafting. Dermatol Clin 1990;8(3):523–37.

[16] Chajchir A, Benzaquen I, Arellano A. [Comparative study on lipoinjection and other methods]. Med Cutan Ibero Lat Am 1988;16(6):489–96. [in Spanish].

[17] Silkiss RZ, Baylis HI. Autogenous fat grafting by injection. Ophthal Plast Reconstr Surg 1987;3(2):71–5.

[18] Illouz YG. Surgical remodeling of the silhouette by aspiration lipolysis or selective lipectomy. Aesthetic Plast Surg 1985;9(1):7–21.

[19] Goldwyn RM. Unproven treatment: whose benefit, whose responsibility? Plast Reconstr Surg 1988;81(6):946–7.

[20] Fredricks S. Fat grafting injection for soft-tissue aumgenation [discussion]. Plast Reconstr Surg 1989;84:935.

[21] Ellenbogen R. Invited commentary on autologus fat injection. Ann Plast Surg 1990;24:297.

[22] Ersek RA. Transplantation of purified autologous fat: a 3-year follow-up is disappointing. Plast Reconstr Surg 1991;87(2):219–27.

[23] Ersek RA, Chang P, Salisbury MA. Lipo layering of autologous fat: an improved technique with promising results. Plast Reconstr Surg 1998;101(3):820–6.

[24] Ellenbogen R, Motykie G, Youn A, et al. Facial reshaping using less invasive methods. Aesthetic Surgery Journal 2005;25(2):144–52.

[25] Coleman SR. Long-term survival of fat transplants: controlled demonstrations. Aesthetic Plast Surg 1995;19(5):421–5.

[26] Guerrerosantos J. Long-term outcome of autologous fat transplantation in aesthetic facial recontouring: sixteen years of experience with 1936 cases. Clin Plast Surg 2000;27(4):515–43.

[27] Trepsat F. Periorbital rejuvenation combining fat grafting and blepharoplasties. Aesthetic Plast Surg 2003;27(4):243–53.

[28] Coleman S. Hand rejuvenation with structural fat grafting. Plast Reconstr Surg 2002;110(7):1731–43.

[29] Coleman S. Structural fat grafting. St Louis (MO): Quality Medical Pub; 2004.

[30] Coleman SR. Structural fat grafting. In: Nahai F, editor. The art of aesthetic surgery: principles & techniques. St Louis (MO): Quality Medical Pub; 2005. p. 289–363.

[31] Rohrich RJ, Sorokin ES, Brown SA. In search of improved fat transfer viability: a quantitative analysis of the role of centrifugation and harvest site. Plast Reconstr Surg 2004;113(1):391–5.

[32] Ullmann Y, Shoshani O, Fodor A, et al. Searching for the favorable donor site for fat injection: in vivo study using the nude mice model. Dermatol Surg 2005;31(10):1304–7.

[33] Coleman SR. Avoidance of arterial occlusion from injection of soft tissue fillers. Aesthetic Surgery Journal 2002;22(6):555–7.

[34] Posten W, Wrone DA, Dover JS, et al. Low-level laser therapy for wound healing: mechanism

and efficacy. Dermatol Surg 2005;31(3):334–40.

[35] Kinney BM. Pulsed Electromagnetic Field Therapy in Plastic Surgery. Aesthetic Surg Journal 2005;25(1):87–92.

[36] Kanchwala SK, Holloway L, Bucky LP. Reliable soft tissue augmentation: a clinical comparison of injectable soft-tissue fillers for facial-volume augmentation. Ann Plast Surg 2005;55(1):30–5 [discussion 35].

[37] Coleman SR. Facial recontouring with lipostructure. Clin Plast Surg 1997;24(2):347–67.

[38] Coleman SR. Problems, Complications and Postprocedure Care: Chapter 4. Structural fat grafting. St. Louis, Mo.: Quality Medical Pub.; 2004. 75–102.

[39] Coleman SR. Infraorbital and Cheek Regions Chapter 11. Structural fat grafting. St. Louis, Mo.: Quality Medical Pub.; 2004. 293–352.

[40] Coleman SR. The technique of periorbital lipoinfiltration. Operative Techniques in Plastic and Reconstructive Surgery 1994;1:20–6.

[41] Coleman SR. Supraorbital area: brow, upper eyelids, and temples. In: Coleman S, editor. Structural fat grafting. St Louis (MO): Quality Medical Pub; 2004. p. 353–400.

[42] Coleman SR. Lips. In: Coleman S, editor. Structural fat grafting. St Louis (MO): Quality Medical Pub; 2004. p. 203–36.

[43] Coleman SR. Lipoinfiltration of the upper lip white roll. Aesthetic Surgery Journal 1994; 14(4):231–4.

[44] Coleman SR. Chin and jawline. In: Coleman S, editor. Structural fat grafting. St Louis (MO): Quality Medical Pub; 2004. p. 237–70.

[45] Coleman SR. Structural fat grafts: the ideal filler? Clin Plast Surg 2001;28(1):111–9.

[46] Orentreich DS, Orentreich N. Subcutaneous incisionless (subcision) surgery for the correction of depressed scars and wrinkles. Dermatol Surg 1995;21(6):543–9.

[47] Coleman SR. Structural fat grafting: more than a permanent filler. Plast Reconstr Surg 2006; 118(3 Suppl):108S–20S.

ELSEVIER
SAUNDERS

CLINICS IN PLASTIC SURGERY

Clin Plastic Surg 33 (2006) 579–586

Vascularized Fat Transfer

Jeffrey D. Friedman, MD[a,*], Farah Khan, MD[b]

Although a rare disorder, Romberg's disease is particularly devastating because it affects previously healthy individuals in their first or second decade of life. Characterized by a progressive atrophy of the facial skin and subcutaneous tissues, Romberg's disease leads to severe facial asymmetry. The progression of the atrophy may last anywhere from 2 to 10 years and initially starts at the maxilla or nasolabial fold and typically progresses to include the angle of the mouth, the cheek, the eyes, the brow, or the ear. Afterwards, it enters a stable phase but, unfortunately, it is often difficult to predict the extent of facial damage because its course varies from individual to individual. Usually, only one side of the face is affected but in rare cases the entire face may be involved [1]. In patients who are affected during the first decade of life, the disease may be more severe because it interferes with the development of the bony skeletal structures [2]. While there is no cure for this disease, nor any treatment that can halt its progression, the goal of surgical treatment once the completion of the disease course is achieved is to help restore a symmetrical facial contour.

Similarly, patients with hemifacial microsomia desire restoration of facial contours and symmetry. Often referred to as first and second branchial arch syndrome, hemifacial microsomia is thought to occur as a result of focal hemorrhage, or a disruption of the blood supply, early during development [3]. While its course also varies from individual to individual, the most common symptoms include microtia, facial palsy, parotid and cheek soft tissue deficiency, and mandibular hypoplasia [4]. The best approach toward management of this disease is a multidisciplinary team approach, with correction of both bony and soft tissue defects. Conventional craniofacial surgery, however, has mostly focused on skeletal correction with maxillary or mandibular osteotomies, bone repositioning, bone grafting, and standard orthognathic surgery [5,6]. We have also found that the combined, staged approach to both the skeletal and soft tissue deficiencies provides the most optimal results. Typically this involves correction of the mandibular deformity as a first procedure. In most cases of severe hemifacial microsomia, the use of mandibular distraction and orthodontics provides the necessary framework for subsequent soft tissue correction. At the completion of the bony reconstruction, soft tissue augmentation can then be performed using either free tissue transfers or autologous nonvascularized fat grafts.

Principles of soft tissue correction

With the realization that skeletal correction does not always improve the perceived volume of the overlying soft tissues, soft tissue reconstruction has gained more attention and undergone much improvement over the past 2 decades. Musculocutaneous flaps,

[a] Institute for Reconstructive Surgery, The Methodist Hospital, Houston, Texas, USA
[b] Division of Plastic Surgery, University of South Florida, Tampa, FL, USA
* Corresponding author.
E-mail address: jfriedman@tmh.tmc.edu (J.D. Friedman).

doi:10.1016/j.cps.2006.09.003
plasticsurgery.theclinics.com

muscle flaps, fasciocutaneous flaps, and free composite tissue transfers have all been used to reconstruct soft tissue facial defects [7]. Although muscle flaps are readily available and relatively simple to harvest, the unpredictability of muscle atrophy over time makes these transfers much less reliable for soft tissue augmentation. Nonvascularized transfers, including dermal fat grafting, large volume fat injections, and silicone implants, have also been used but the results have been inconsistent [8]. When favorable conditions exist, however (eg, ample available donor fat, well-vascularized recipient bed, and a supple overlying skin envelope), favorable results can be obtained using these traditional techniques (Fig. 1). Alternatively, given the greater predictability of vascularized transfers and keeping

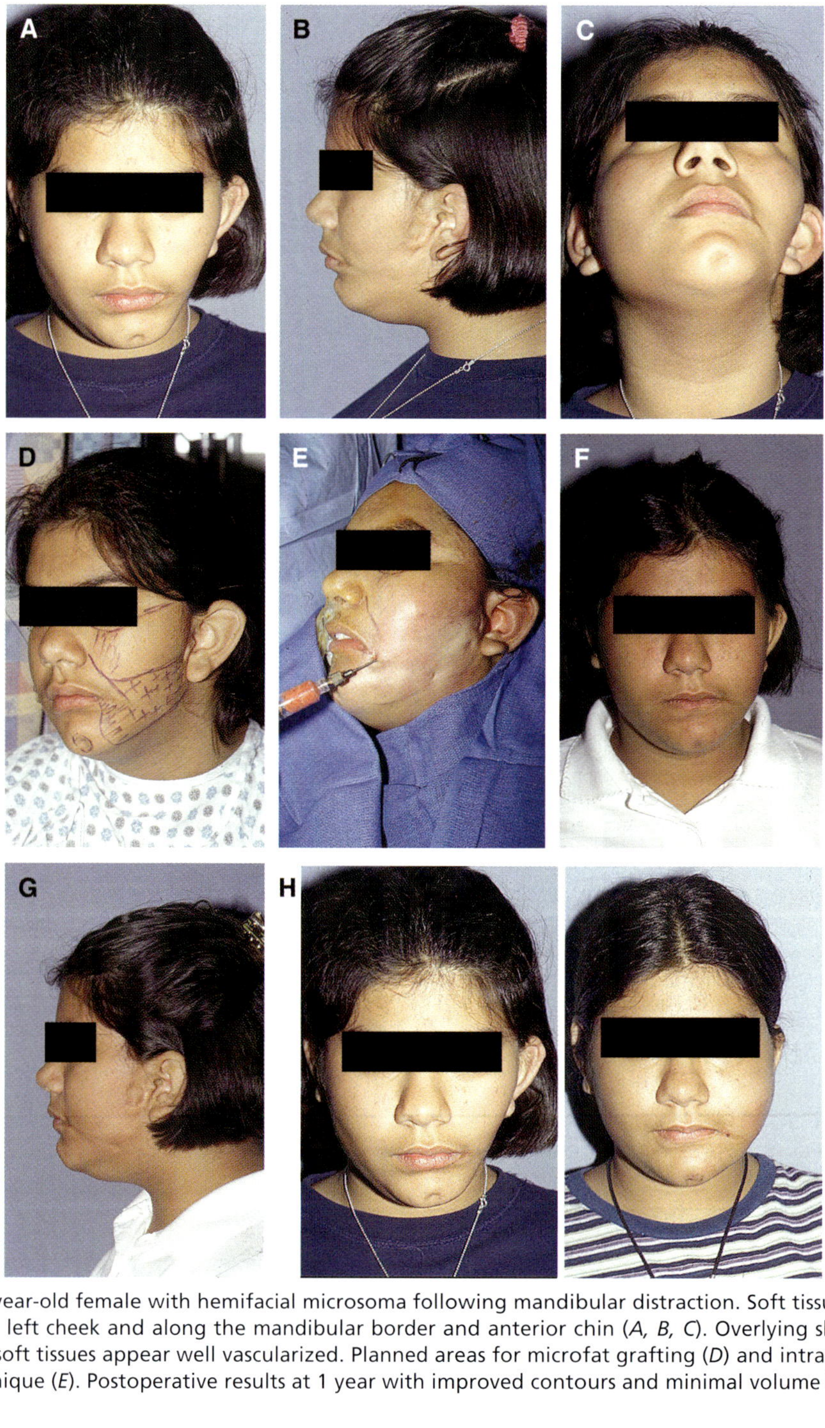

Fig. 1. A 13-year-old female with hemifacial microsoma following mandibular distraction. Soft tissue deficiency noted in the left cheek and along the mandibular border and anterior chin (*A, B, C*). Overlying skin envelope and deeper soft tissues appear well vascularized. Planned areas for microfat grafting (*D*) and intraoperative injection technique (*E*). Postoperative results at 1 year with improved contours and minimal volume loss (*F, G, H*).

the reconstructive philosophy of replacing "like with like" in mind, free vascularized dermal-fat flaps have gained much greater acceptance for the restoration of large soft tissue defects in these congenital anomalies, traumatic injuries, and progressive hemifacial atrophy.

While the obvious goal is to achieve optimal cosmesis, an adequate soft tissue bed is often necessary to protect an underlying bone graft or to provide complete coverage of an implant [8]. Additionally, the relative vascularity of the recipient bed may also influence the type of reconstruction chosen. Certainly, when the inherent blood supply to the facial area is compromised (postradiation, multiple previous operative procedures, Romberg's atrophy), microfat grafts and dermal fat grafts are much less likely to be successful. In such cases additional vascularity can be transferred to the area with the use of free fasciocutaneous flaps. A variety of such donor sites have been described and used for many years. These include the free deltopectoral flap [9], groin flap [10], and scapular and parascapular flaps [11]. Newer methods have included the customized parascapular flap [12] and deep inferior epigastric perforator flap [13]. All of these methods have advantages and disadvantages and no one method has emerged as the best possible option for all scenarios.

The free deltopectoral dermal-fat flap was the first free tissue transfer used to treat hemifacial atrophy patients [9]. Unfortunately, the wide donor site deformity was often unacceptable, especially in young patients. This led to the introduction and the use of the free groin flap in large part because the donor scar is easily concealed in the bathing suit area. Although preferred by some surgeons, it has rarely been used in our practice for various reasons. In many cases the groin flap can be rather bulky and may require staged debulking. The pedicle vessels, the superficial circumflex iliac artery (SCIA) and vein, are relatively small thus making microvascular anastomoses technically challenging. These vessels also course in the deep layer of the subcutaneous tissue and, therefore, very careful debulking is necessary to avoid damage to the vessel at the time of initial thinning and contouring of the flap [14]. Secondary debulking procedures can also lead to scar tissue formation and subcutaneous fibrosis of the face. In addition, the donor scar may now be unacceptable to many females because of the recent changes in fashion and clothing, thus making the scar more visible than it has been in the past.

Scapular and parascapular free tissue transfers

The use of the scapular and parascapular flaps for facial contour restoration was reported by both Stern and colleagues [15] and Upton and colleagues [11] in 1992. Based on the circumflex scapular arteries, large volumes of well-vascularized soft tissue can be harvested. In addition, the circumflex scapular vessels can usually be dissected more proximally to the thoracodorsal pedicle, which affords greater pedicle length as well as increased vessel diameter thus making the microsurgical anastomoses technically easier. In those cases where the temporal vessels and the facial vessels are unavailable for anastomosis, the thoracodorsal vessels tend to have a better size match for those in the upper neck. Unfortunately however, these flaps originally included large skin paddles in their design, which often led to hypertrophic and unsightly scars.

Not long after, Longaker and Siebert [7] and Siebert and colleagues [12] introduced the concept of a customized parascapular flap that incorporated numerous fascial extensions at the periphery of the transfer. Unlike the traditional parascapular flap, the dorsal thoracic fascia could be incorporated into this flap design to satisfy thin tissue defects. Folded into multiple layers, dorsal thoracic fascial extensions can correct even the most difficult soft tissue deformities around the eye, nose, upper lip, and chin [12]. According to Siebert and Longaker, this flap is "reliable, less bulky than muscle flaps, and yields predictable long-term results without accompanying muscle atrophy." In addition, given the anatomic position of the circumflex vessels along the deep boarder of the flap, the superficial soft tissue can be contoured to any desired thickness based on the volume requirements of the individual patient.

The use of the word customized for this flap is truly indicative of its composition because even the lateral border of the scapula with bony lengths up to 15 cm can be included in the flap design for simultaneous mandibular reconstruction. The donor site can also be oriented in any direction as long as the vascular pedicle is taken at the point it enters the flap. This variability has important implications for donor vessel selection in that it allows easy access to both the temporal and facial vessels. If more bulk is necessary, it can be obtained by harvesting parts of local, regional muscles such as the teres major or more commonly may include both the transverse-oriented scapular flap with the more obliquely oriented parascapular skin paddle [12].

Operative technique

The obvious goal for free flap reconstruction of the face is to accurately provide soft tissue to those areas that are volume deficient. Essential to this process are the preoperative markings. It is important to mark the patient in the upright position and accurately outline those areas that are soft tissue deficient and to delineate the degree to which these areas require augmentation. Based on these markings, a template, fashioned from x-ray film, can be created that will be used when harvesting the flap from the back (Fig. 2).

In most cases, the recipient site is dissected through a limited preauricular incision to obtain optimal cosmesis. This incision can be carried up into the temporal scalp should the superficial temporal vessels be used for anastomosis. Conversely, when the facial vessels are more favorable, a separate transverse submandibular incision can be used. Siebert and colleagues [12] prefer to use the superficial temporal artery and vein and have found them to be adequate in diameter for microvascular anastomoses in 35 of 60 consecutive cases. While the anatomy of the superficial temporal artery is quite constant and presents a reasonable size match for the circumflex vessels, the superficial temporal vein has a more variable anatomy having one, two, or even three branches [16]. Imanishi and colleagues [16] found that in 11 of 15 specimens, the course of the superficial temporal vein varied from that of the superficial temporal artery. In five specimens, the superficial temporal vein bifurcated and became two major branches: frontal and parietal. In three specimens, the superficial temporal vein became one major branch and in the other three specimens, the parietal branch bifurcated and became two major branches after the frontal branch was given off. This variability is what often causes the superficial temporal vein to be less than optimal for microvascular anastomosis and, in our experience, the vein may be completely absent thus obviating its use. In cases where the superficial temporal vessels are inadequate, the incision may need to be extended down into the neck to allow for anastomosis to branches of the external carotid artery and accompanying veins or to the facial vessels via a separate incision [12]. Preoperative Doppler examination may be helpful in determining which vessels are most favorable.

The preauricular incision also allows for the necessary elevation of the facial flap. The facial skin is elevated in the subcutaneous plane to the extent dictated by the template. Dissection extends slightly beyond this point so that the flap can be tapered in these areas and a smooth transition can be created between the flap and the native soft tissues. Once this has been accomplished and the donor vessels have been dissected and prepared, attention is then directed to the back where the flap is elevated. Again the template is used to assist in determining the dimensions of the flap to be elevated. As is true of most free tissue transfers, as much pedicle length as possible is desired. This is obtained by dissecting the circumflex vessels between the teres major and teres minor as noted previously (Fig. 3).

If the patient is placed in the lateral decubitus position at the beginning of the procedure, flap dissection and microvascular anatomoses can be performed without necessitating a position change. Despite such, it is usually best to place the patient in the supine position so that symmetry can be assessed at the time of flap inset. This is accomplished by securing the distal margins of the flap into the peripheral margins of the subcutaneous dissection. This is best accomplished by using horizontal mattress sutures placed transcutaneously. These sutures are then tied over dental rolls so that excessive pressure on the elevated skin flaps can be avoided. The flap can be thinned as needed; however, there is little need for overcorrection since there is minimal soft tissue atrophy following this procedure so

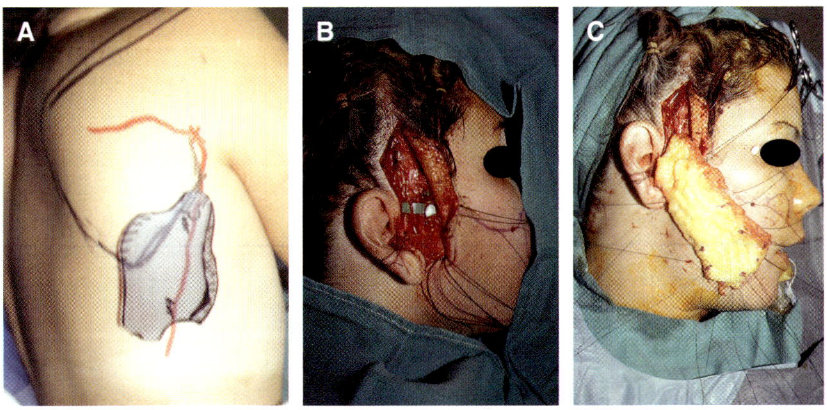

Fig. 2. A template is made using x-ray film and patterned from the area of soft tissue deficiency. Dissection of the recipient vessels is then performed, which will allow proper orientation of the flap (*A*). A parascapular flap is then raised to include an area of soft tissue equivalent to that of the facial defect (*B*). The flap is then harvested and oriented to conform to the soft tissue deficit (*C*). Microvascular anastomoses are then performed.

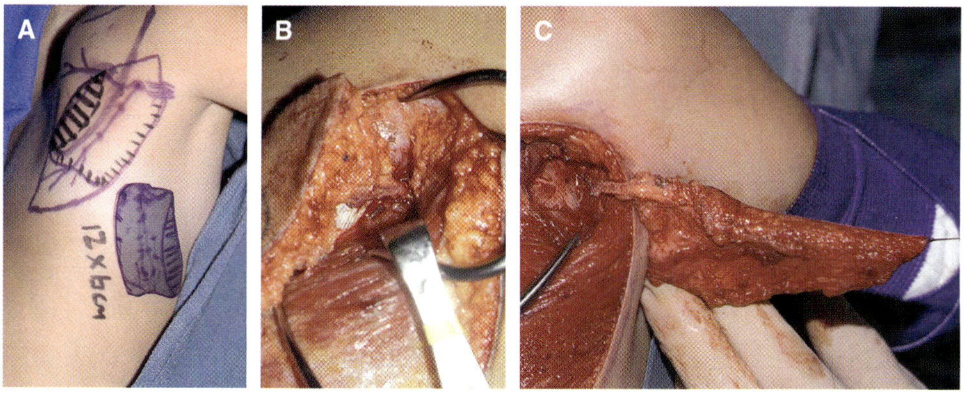

Fig. 3. The template is used to delineate the extent of dissection as well as the variable thicknesses needed within the flap (*A*). The circumflex scapular vessels emerge from between the teres major and teres minor muscles (*B*) and are then dissected further anteriorly to achieve greater pedicle length and diameter (*C*).

long as the microvascular repair remains patent. A suction drain is then placed and the wounds are closed in layers. Should there be significant tension on the flaps as a result of skin closure, consideration should be given to leaving some portion of the skin incisions open and plan to close these secondarily. We have found the use of intraoperative steroids helpful in the early reduction of facial swelling in these patients.

Postoperative care is relatively straightforward. Patients are instructed to keep the head of their beds elevated and avoid any significant exertion for 7 to 10 days. Sutures are removed at a week following surgery and patients are allowed to return to their usual activities at 3 weeks postoperatively.

Because of the limited preauricular incision primarily used with the customized parascapular flap, the most common postoperative complication is a hematoma. Obtaining meticulous hemostasis is difficult because of the limited visualization of the facial midline and the excellent blood supply to the facial area. In the experience of Siebert and colleagues [12], hematomas have not compromised their final reconstructive results and the cosmetic advantage of the limited incision outweighs the possibility of a limited hematoma. Furthermore, the recent use of endoscopic instrumentation has drastically improved the visualization of this area with the flap inset and thus allows for better hemostasis.

Results from this form of reconstruction remain quite satisfying. In many cases dramatic improvement in facial contour can be achieved, often with a single operation (Fig. 4). These operations remain far from perfect however. As with any operative procedure, further improvement can often be obtained with minor revision procedures. In our experience these have usually involved microfat grafting to medial areas of the face that were not fully corrected (Fig. 5). Areas of overcorrection can be remedied with direct excision of the excess fat in the affected

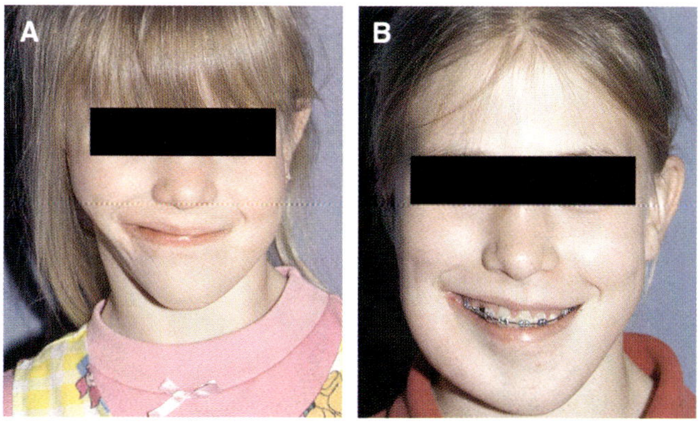

Fig. 4. A 7-year-old female following mandibular distraction with a severe form of hemifacial microsomia (*A*). Three years postoperatively demonstrating permanence of the soft tissue correction using a parascapular free tissue transfer (*B*).

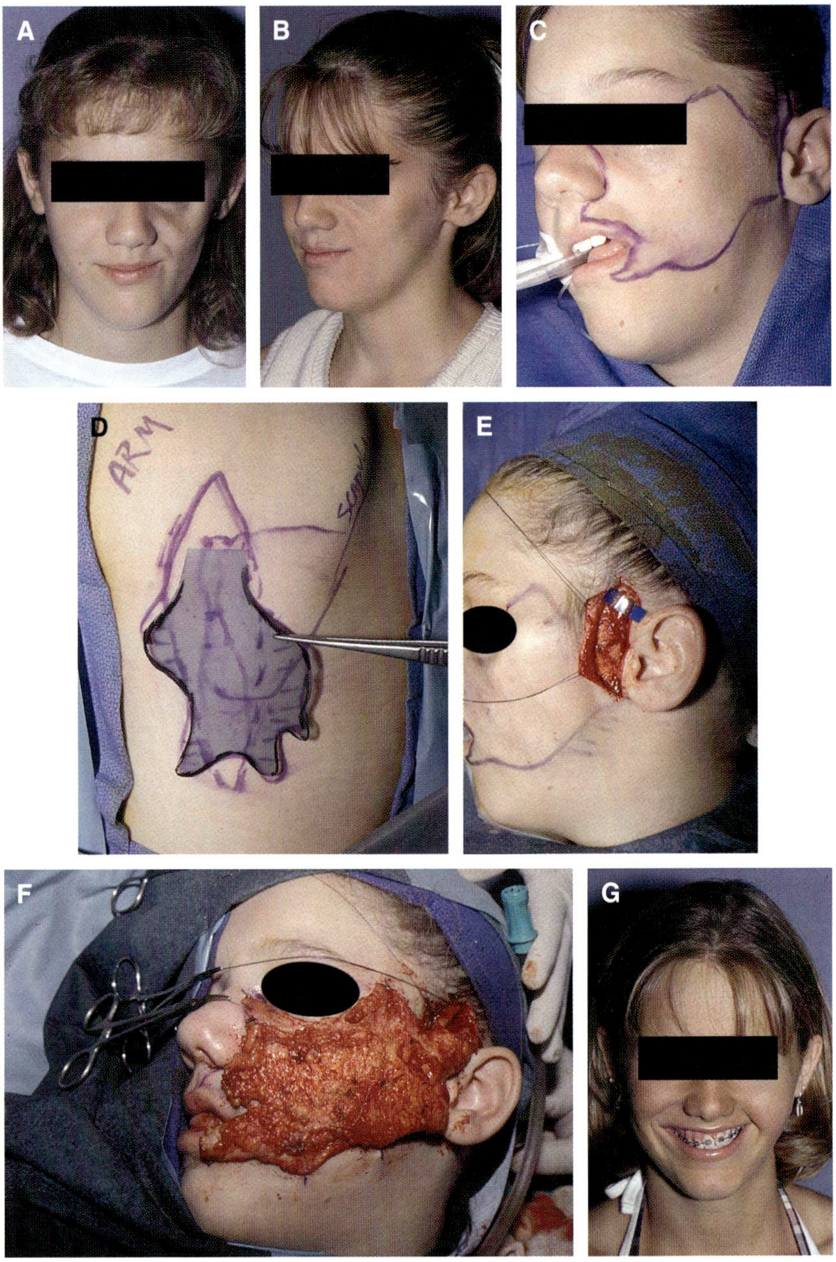

Fig. 5. A 13-year-old female with Romberg's disease with stable soft tissue atrophy for 3 years (*A, B*). Plan for soft tissue fill (*C*), which was achieved with a parascapular free flap anastomosed to the superficial temporal vessels (*D, E*). Flap and inset and 3-year postoperative result. Microfat grafts were necessary for volume restoration to the upper lip (*F, G*).

area. These procedures can often be performed in the outpatient setting. Over time, gravity may also influence the final appearance of these flaps. In some cases, the flap may settle inferiorly, thus creating a visible junction of the flap with the native cheek skin (Fig. 6). This can also be corrected with a combination of micrografting and, if needed, some reduction in the volume of the flap in the superior aspect. Elevation of the facial skin much in the way as a facelift may also be necessary and is simply performed.

Recent advances

While the customized parascapular flap seems to be the most frequently used flap for the correction of facial asymmetry [14], hypertrophic scarring at the donor site has been reported in some patients. In

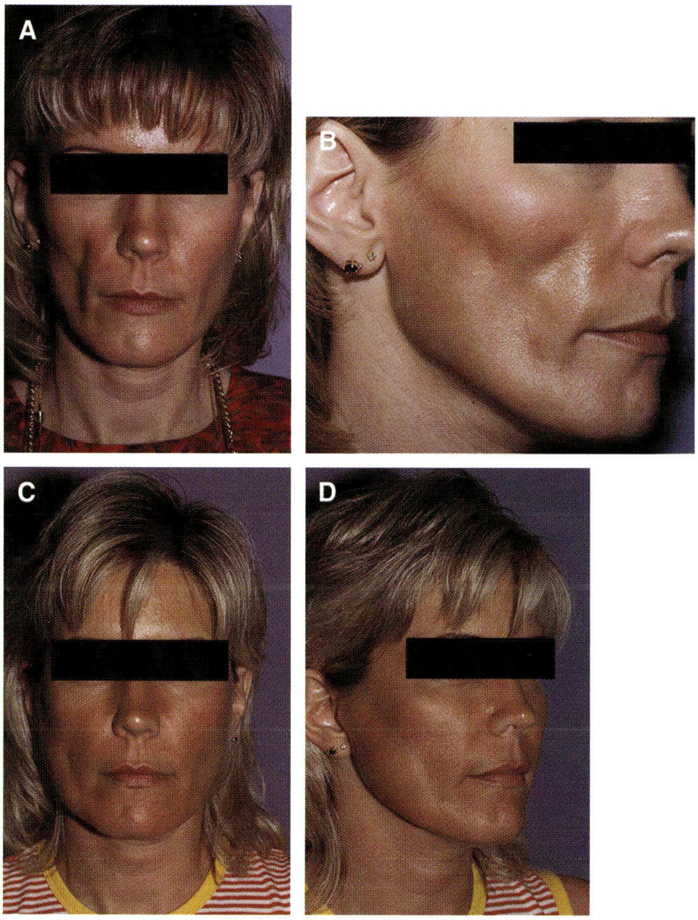

Fig. 6. A middle-aged female with Romberg's atrophy involving the central cheek (*A, B*). Postoperative result at 1 year with some inferior settling of the flap and a distinct junction between the flap and native cheek soft tissues (*C, D*). Future revisions including microfat grafting and improved fixation to the SMAS may alleviate this appearance.

addition, because of the donor site's proximity to the face, a positioning change is sometimes necessary, adding more time to completing the flap transfer and, hence, becoming a significant disadvantage [13].

Abdominal flaps, such as the superficial inferior epigastric artery (SIEA) flap and the deep inferior epigastric perforator flap (DIEP), have also been used to improve facial contour. While the SIEA flap is truly noninvasive and offers sufficient bulk and an easily hidden donor-site scar, its variable anatomy and short vascular pedicle are often problematic. Use of the DIEP flap is more reliable because it has a long vascular pedicle and still leaves the rectus muscles intact. Unfortunately, a longer operating time and the unavoidable sagging associated with this flap are significant disadvantages. Therefore, Koshima and colleagues [14] advocate the use of a customized DIEP flap: the paraumbilical adiposal flap with one-stage removal of bulky fatty tissue. This flap, referred to as a perforator flap, is elevated from the lower portion of the umbilicus based on a single, main paraumbilical perforator. Although the dissection is challenging, a significant amount of the superficial fatty layer can be easily removed. This prevents the flap from developing hard subcutaneous tissue, fat necrosis, which results in scar formation at the recipient site.

To further improve cosmesis, Koshima and colleagues [14] advocate the use of an intraoral approach instead of a limited preauricular incision to access the recipient site. An intraoral incision is made to create a subcutaneous pocket in the cheek region for flap transfer. This pocket is created subperiosteally on the maxillary and zygomatic bones and may be extended if a subcutaneous pocket in the mandibular region is needed. The facial vessels are used as the recipient vessels and are exposed through a small skin incision in the submandibular region. This space is then extended upward to join with the subcutaneous cheek pocket for passage of the flap vascular pedicle.

The major advantages of this flap are that it leaves minimum donor site morbidity and allows for one-stage reconstruction because it can be debulked primarily. Furthermore, the use of an intraoral approach allows for a "scarless" operation. To overcome the sagging inherent with dermal fat flaps placed under the dermis, an intraoral approach even allows for the placement of the flap in the subperiosteal space. Because the periosteum anchors the flap, it may prevent drooping of the fatty tissue [14]. The primary disadvantage of this flap is that it requires meticulous dissecting technique at the donor site and has a short vascular pedicle. With adequate training, however, this challenge can be overcome.

Summary

The use of free tissue transfers has dramatically improved the outcomes of soft tissue reconstructions of the face. This is particularly true when large volumes of soft tissue are needed or when the recipient bed has a compromised local blood supply. Although traditional fat grafting procedures often allow for satisfactory results in some patients, the use of scapular and parascapular free tissue transfers has markedly improved the predictability of these reconstructions, often in a single stage. As perforator flap reconstructions evolve over time, these types of flaps may eventually supplant the available fasciocutaneous free flaps as the flap of choice in these reconstructions primarily because of improved donor site scarring and morbidity.

References

[1] National Institute of Neurological Disorders and Stroke, National Institutes of Health. NINDS Parry-Romberg Information Page. Available at: http://www.ninds.nih.gov/disorders/parry_romberg/parry_romberg.htm.

[2] Inigo F, Jimenez-Murat Y, Arroya O, et al. Restoration of facial contour in Romberg's disease and hemifacial microsomia: experience with 118 cases. Microsurg 2000;20:167–72.

[3] National Craniofacial Association. Hemifacial microsomia. Available at: http://www.faces-cranio.org/Disord/Hemi.htm.

[4] Converse JM, Coccaro PJ, Becker M, et al. On hemifacial microsomia. The first and second branchial arch syndrome. Plast Reconstr Surg 1973;51:268–79.

[5] Kaban L, Moses M, Mulliken J. Surgical correction of hemifacial microsomia in the growing child. Plast Reconstr Surg 1988;82:9–19.

[6] Murray J, Kaban L, Mulliken J. Analysis and treatment of hemifacial microsomia. Plast Reconstr Surg 1984;74:186–99.

[7] Longaker M, Siebert J. Microsurgical correction of facial contour in congenital craniofacial malformations: the marriage of hard and soft tissue. Plast Reconstr Surg 1996;98:942–50.

[8] Ji Y, Li T, Shamburger S, et al. Microsurgical anterolateral thigh fasciocutaneous flap for facial contour correction in patients with hemifacial microsomia. Microsurg 2002;22:34–8.

[9] Fujino T, Tanino R, Sugimoto C. Microvascular transfer of free deltopectoral dermal-fat flap. Plast Reconstr Surg 1975;55:428–34.

[10] Harashina T, Nakajima T, Yoshimura Y. A free groin flap reconstruction in progressive facial hemi-atrophy. Br J Plast Surg 1977;30:14–6.

[11] Upton RE, Mulliken JB, Murray JE. The use of scapular and parascapular flaps for cheek reconstruction. Plast Reconstr Surg 1992;90:959–71.

[12] Siebert JW, Anson G, Longaker M. Microsurgical correction of facial asymmetry in 60 consecutive cases. Plast Reconstr Surg 1996;97:354–63.

[13] Koshima I, Inagawa K, Urushiara K, et al. Deep inferior epigastric perforator dermal-fat or adiposal flap for correction of craniofacial contour deformities. Plast Reconstr Surg 2000;106:10–5.

[14] Koshima I, Urushibara K, Inagawa K, et al. One-stage facial contour augmentation with an intraoral groin adipose flap transfer. Ann Plast Surg 2001;46:450–3.

[15] Stern H, Elliott L, Beegle P. Progressive hemifacial atrophy associated with Lyme disease. Plast Reconstr Surg 1992;90:479–83.

[16] Imanishi N, Nakajima H, Minabe T, et al. Venous drainage architecture of the temporal and parietal regions: anatomy of the superficial temporal artery and vein. Plast Reconstr Surg 2002;109:2197–203.

ELSEVIER
SAUNDERS

CLINICS IN PLASTIC SURGERY

Clin Plastic Surg 33 (2006) 587–596

Collagen-Containing Fillers: Alone and in Combination

Leslie Baumann, MD, FAAD

Collagen, the major structural component of the dermis and the most abundant protein found in humans, is responsible for imparting strength and support to human skin. Loss of collagen with aging and sun exposure leads to skin fragility. In addition, it may play a role in facial flushing in patients who have rosacea and severe photodamage. It is believed that loss of the collagen support surrounding the blood vessels allows the vessels to remain dilated, giving the skin a flushed appearance. Preventing the loss of collagen is the purpose of many skin care topical products and oral supplements. Increasing the amount of skin collagen is the mechanism by which intense pulsed light, dermabrasion, carbon dioxide laser, Fraxel laser, and other technologies treat aged skin. Collagen plays an important role in the prevention, development, and treatment of aged skin.

The dermal matrix in adult human skin is composed primarily of type I collagen (80% to 85%) and type III collagen (10% to 15%). Both types of collagen are produced by dermal fibroblasts as α-procollagens. In the presence of copper and ascorbic acid (vitamin C), prolyl and lysyl hydroxylase add hydroxyl ions to proline and lysyl residues. The alpha chains develop into the triple helix and are then released into the extracellular matrix, where the protocollagens N-proteinase and C-proteinase cleave the amino and carboxy terminal domain of the propeptides. Two α1 chains and one α2 chain constitute the collagen type I triple helices, and three identical α1 chains compose the collagen III triple helices. Once assembled, these collagen molecules mix with noncollagenous molecules to form fibrils.

During the embryonic period of human development, type III collagen (also known as "fetal collagen") outweighs type I collagen in human skin. After birth, however, the ratio changes in favor of type I collagen [1], and it is the latter type that

University of Miami, Miller School of Medicine, 4701 North Meridian Avenue, Suite 7450, Miami Beach, FL 33140, USA
E-mail address: lsb@derm.net

doi:10.1016/j.cps.2006.08.001
plasticsurgery.theclinics.com

predominates during childhood and early adulthood in skin not chronically exposed to the sun. Over time, the structural proteins and key components of the skin diminish, manifesting in skin aging. Epidermal and dermal atrophy, as well as flattening of the rete ridges, characterizes intrinsically or naturally aged skin [2]. Aged fibroblasts produce lower levels of collagen in vivo and in vitro. This diminished output is responsible for the 20% reduction in dermal thickness characteristic of extrinsically aged (photoaged or otherwise environmentally compromised) skin. Epidermal atrophy with thickened, fragmented, and irregular collagen bundles is also typical of extrinsically aged skin [3]. In addition, the proportion of collagen III increases in human skin with age [4]. Collagenase and other matrix metalloproteinases (MMPs) degrade collagen. UV radiation has been demonstrated to raise MMP levels in vivo, thereby increasing collagen degradation and resulting in visible skin aging [5,6]. Furthermore, reduced collagen formation and low levels of type I and III procollagen precursors are characteristic of photodamaged skin, corresponding to the clinical severity of photoaged skin [7,8].

Glycosaminoglycans (GAGs) and elastin are the other major fundamental constituents of the dermal skin that influence its outward appearance. GAGs are polysaccharide chains with repeating disaccharide units attached to a core protein. Situated in cramped areas with a fibrous matrix where cells have little room for movement, GAGs potently bind water, directing it into the skin and leaving it plump, soft, and hydrated. Consequently, these compounds, of which dermatan sulfate and hyaluronic acid (HA), or hyaluronan, are the most prevalent, are believed to assist in maintaining salt and water balance. With age and sun exposure, GAG content is known to diminish.

HA is found in all connective tissue [9], especially in the ground substance of normal dermis, and is diffusely distributed throughout the dermal layer. It plays a significant role in cell growth, membrane receptor function, and adhesion. Stabilizing intercellular structures and generating the elastoviscous matrix for collagen and elastin fibers, binding them together in the proper formation, are the primary functions of this GAG compound [10]. In fact, the viscoelastic and stabilizing qualities, as well as its protective action on cell membranes, render HA the GAG most worthy of interest and use in research and development as a dermal filling agent [9]. Given its capacity to bind water as much as 1000 times its volume, HA strongly affects dermal volume and compressibility [11]. In young skin, HA is found at the periphery of collagen and elastin fibers and at their intersection, but these connections decline with age, theoretically accounting for the disorganized bundles of collagen and elastin fibers seen in aged skin [12].

The skin exhibits recoil capacity, or elasticity, by virtue of its elastic fibers, which are complex extracellular matrix polymers composed of at least 19 different proteins [13]. Elastin fibers, which play a significant role in maintaining skin integrity, build on templates formed by bundles of fibrillin microfibrils. They amass at the periphery of collagen bundles—attached by HA, it is believed [12]. Damage to elastin fibers is believed to account at least partially for the reduced skin elasticity characteristic of aged skin [14]. Manifesting in rhytides, damage to elastin can occur in young people and in the absence of significant extrinsic causes. Defects in elastin fibers were noted in a child with "wrinkled skin syndrome" [15]. Exogenous factors, especially excessive sun exposure, more often cause the degradation of elastin, which appears amorphous under light microscopy. Indeed, photoaged skin is characterized by such "elastosis."

With age, collagen, HA, and elastin levels decline significantly, yielding an older facial appearance. Located between the epidermis and subcutaneous fat, the dermis imparts thickness to the skin. Soft tissue augmentation has the purpose of replacing the primary components of the dermal layer lost through aging so as to achieve a desirable, albeit temporary, cosmetic enhancement, including a younger facial appearance. Manufacturers have achieved great success in devising dermal filling products that can temporarily replace collagen and HA; no such products are yet available that can replace elastin.

Soft tissue augmentation has been a popular therapeutic option as a dermal replacement filler since its inception. In 1893, Neuber [16] became the first physician to transplant fat from the arms into facial defects in humans. Paraffin and silicone, which carried the risk of foreign body granulomas, were subsequently used as injectable fillers. The viability of animal- and human-derived collagen implants for soft tissue augmentation was studied in the 1970s [17]. Through the evolutionary development of filling agents, a general consensus has emerged that the ideal filler substance would be easy to obtain, implant, and store; it would pose no risk for inducing allergic or hypersensitive reactions while yielding a cosmetically desirable result. Such an agent would also be nontoxic, noncarcinogenic, long-lasting, and inexpensive.

Perhaps because of the obvious defect in collagen in aged human skin, collagen derived from both animals and humans became the object of investigation as a soft tissue filler beginning in the 1970s.

Since then, several studies have demonstrated the safety and efficacy of bovine- and human-derived collagen fillers. Injectable collagen implants have become well-established treatment modalities for cosmetic indications and are considered to be the closest to ideal filling agents yet available. The introduction of HA products has widened the array of choices in the soft tissue augmentation armamentarium, but a truly ideal filling substance remains elusive. For this reason, combining two or more different fillers in one procedure may render the best possible correction.

Bovine collagen implants

Zyderm I, Zyderm II, and Zyplast (Allergan Corporation, Irvine, California) are the three types of collagen products derived from bovine dermal collagen. Each of these soft tissue augmentation fillers contains 95% type I collagen and 5% type III collagen. Approved for use in humans by the US Food and Drug Administration (FDA) in 1981, Zyderm I contains 3.5% bovine dermal collagen suspended in physiologic phosphate-buffered sodium chloride solution and 0.3% lidocaine. Zyderm II, approved by the FDA in 1983, is composed of 6.5% bovine dermal collagen as well as 0.3% lidocaine. Approved by the FDA in 1985, Zyplast is composed of 3.5% bovine dermal collagen cross-linked with 0.0075% glutaraldehyde, which reinforces the collagen fibers and prolongs the overall duration of the correction. All three products are prepared in 0.5- to 1.5-mL preloaded syringes and must be kept refrigerated until use.

Indications for Zyderm I and II include correction of superficial facial rhytides, such as glabellar lines, horizontal forehead lines, crow's feet, fine perioral lines, and scars [18]. Zyderm II is more suitable for moderate to deep wrinkles because it contains more collagen. Deeper lines, such as nasolabial folds, atrophic scars (eg, deep post-acne, past traumatic, postviral, postoperative), and the vermilion border of the lips, are among the indications for Zyplast [18]. Correction with bovine collagen fillers is temporary. Generally, the cosmetic enhancement from these products lasts approximately 3 months before collagenase succeeds in degrading the filler [19]. Some reports indicate that bovine collagen filler has lasted as long as 18 months, but this is not common [20]. Zyplast lasts longer than either Zyderm product [21]. Differences among the products are not the only factors influencing correction duration. The amount of implant used, the treatment area selected, and injection techniques all affect the longevity of the correction. Overcorrection is necessary to achieve an optimal cosmetic result. Because Zyderm and Zyplast contain lidocaine, the treatment area is partially anesthetized, typically obviating the use of additional numbing agents. Topical lidocaine, and less frequently nerve blocks, may be used to reduce the pain of injection for patients experiencing pain from the standard procedure.

Although they are uncommon, there are two types of adverse reactions, nonhypersensitive and hypersensitive (or allergic), to the injection of bovine-derived collagen implants. The typical nonhypersensitive reactions include abscesses, bacterial infections, beading, cyst formation, ecchymoses, herpes virus infection, and local necrosis. Several of these reactions may be prevented or easily treated. Antiviral medications will help prevent episodes or eruptions of the herpes virus. To minimize the risk for bruising, patients should be instructed to avoid taking nonsteroidal anti-inflammatory drugs, aspirin, vitamin E, and anticoagulants, if possible, for 10 days before the scheduled procedure. To reduce the risk for inducing local necrosis, care should be taken to avoid injecting Zyplast into the glabellar region [22].

Hypersensitive or allergic reactions to the introduction or injection of foreign substances are also possible in patients treated with bovine collagen agents. It is believed that approximately 3% of the general population is sensitive to bovine collagen [23]. To reduce the likelihood of eliciting an allergic reaction, the recommended protocol before bovine collagen injection is to perform two consecutive skin tests 6 weeks and 2 weeks before the scheduled treatment. Injected subcutaneously on the volar aspect of the forearm, the skin test contains 0.3 mL of Zyderm I in a prefilled tuberculin syringe [24]. Failure to react to the two skin tests suggests that a patient is unlikely to react to the bovine collagen implant. After one negative test, the risk for allergy remains between 1.3% and 6.2% [25,26]; it is 0.5% after two negative tests. Rarely, allergic reaction may occur after multiple treatments. If a hypersensitive reaction arises in a patient treated several times, the patient should be instructed to monitor the site between 48 and 72 hours after the implant is introduced and to make an appointment to see the treating physician 4 weeks after the procedure.

It is important to communicate clearly to patients who have hypersensitivity reactions to bovine collagen that such responses typically resolve within 4 to 24 months [27,28]. Hypersensitive reactions to bovine collagen agents may be treated with topical, intralesional, or a brief course of systemic corticosteroids. Allergic reactions to bovine collagen have reportedly been treated with success with oral cyclosporine [29] and topical tacrolimus [30].

Some authors have suggested that bovine collagen may induce an autoimmune reaction, notably dermatomyositis, in patients receiving this injectable filler [31]. However, the incident rate of polymyositis/dermatomyositis in patients who received bovine collagen was no higher than that in the control-matched population in a study conducted by Hanke and colleagues [32]. Other reports point to the low likelihood that patients will develop autoimmune disorders as a result of injection with bovine collagen [33,34].

Other forms of bovine collagen

Artecoll (Artes Medical USA, San Diego, CA) is an agent composed of polymethylmethacrylate microspheres (PMMA) suspended in bovine collagen and lidocaine. Because PMMA is nonbiodegradable, the intended augmentation or correction is rendered more durable after the collagen is absorbed in the body [35]. As with Zyderm and Zyplast, a pretreatment skin test is required before injection, because this substance is also derived from bovine material. Artecoll has been used to treat facial wrinkles, as well as for lip, chin, and malar augmentation [35]. Correction effects lasting as long as 1 year have been reported among patients treated with Artecoll [36]. ArteFill (Artes Medical USA, San Diego, CA), the next-generation derivative of Artecoll, which is composed of PMMA suspended in a 3.5% solution of bovine collagen containing 0.3% lidocaine, is expected to attain in late 2006 the mantle of the only permanent filler approved by the FDA (that will also be available globally) [37]. By volume, ArteFill is 20% PMMA and 80% bovine collagen, with the microspheres acting as structural scaffolding to support the much larger volume of connective tissue deposition that replaces the injected collagen [38].

Human-derived bioengineered collagen

The risk of provoking hypersensitive reactions is associated with all bovine-derived dermal fillers. For this reason, human bioengineered collagen and HA-containing products have been developed and have subsequently become the most popular fillers in the United States.

CosmoDerm and CosmoPlast

Approved by the FDA in March 2003, CosmoDerm I, CosmoDerm II, and CosmoPlast (Allergan Corporation, Irvine, California) are human-based collagen implants that contain type I and III human collagen. These agents are produced when dermal fibroblasts are harvested from bioengineered human skin cells, placed into a three-dimensional mesh, and cultured in a bioreactor that simulates the human body. Nutritionally supported by the medium, the dermal fibroblasts synthesize collagen and extracellular matrix proteins.

CosmoDerm I is composed of 35 mg/mL of human-derived collagen dispersed in a phosphate-based saline solution and 0.3% lidocaine. The collagen concentration in CosmoDerm II doubles the collagen concentration contained in CosmoDerm I. CosmoPlast has the same ingredients as these products but is cross-linked by glutaraldehyde, rendering it more resistant to degradation and hence more suitable for deeper placement or correction.

Superficial wrinkles are the primary indications for CosmoDerm. Because it displays a stiff consistency, even more so than HA-containing agents, CosmoPlast is ideal for the vermilion border of the lips, the bridge of the nose, and deeper furrows, as well as to raise the corners of the mouth. CosmoPlast is typically used to treat medium and deep wrinkles in combination with an HA filler, with the HA product used second and injected into the same planes as the collagen filler. Skin testing is not required for any of the human-derived collagen products, which makes their use more appealing to many patients. In addition, the sole and rarely seen adverse reactions associated with these products have been bruising, erythema, and swelling. The risk for bruising may be mitigated by the platelet-aggregating effects believed to be exhibited by the collagen in CosmoDerm and CosmoPlast [39,40]. Furthermore, the inclusion of lidocaine in these products reduces the risk for swelling and bruising by inhibiting the activation of eosinophils [40]. These products, like Zyderm and Zyplast, must be kept refrigerated. The cosmetic effects of CosmoDerm and CosmoPlast are immediate. Longevity trials have not been performed. However, the general consensus is that CosmoDerm lasts approximately 3 months, and CosmoPlast injections, contingent on the treatment area, injection technique, and amount of filling agent used, last about 4 to 7 months [41]. CosmoDerm and CosmoPlast are contraindicated in patients who are allergic to lidocaine.

Hyaluronic acid products

Filling agents derived from HA pose reduced risk of inducing allergy and immunogenicity, because HA is chemically identical across all species [42]. In fact, because HA occurs naturally in all cells in all species, skin tests are not required when using these products. Consequently, HA fillers may be used during a patient's first visit. In addition, injected HA imparts volume to water by means of binding, allowing muscles and joints to glide smoothly, and it is metabolized to carbon dioxide and water.

At this time, no lidocaine-containing HA fillers are on the market, but several are being studied. HA has a low pH, so stinging on injection may occur. In addition, HA has a heparin-like effect that can lead to an increased incidence of bruising as compared with collagen-containing fillers.

Hylaform or Hylan B

Hylaform, also known as Hylan B (Allergan Corporation, Irvine, California), is derived from rooster combs, which contain copious amounts of HA. HAs derived from a rooster source have longer chains than those derived from a bacterial source, which gives them distinctive characteristics one should keep in mind when choosing a filler. This injectable filler, which was approved by the FDA for cosmetic use on April 22, 2004, is created by introducing sulfonyl-bis-ethyl cross-links between hydroxyl groups of the polysaccharide chains of hyaluronan [43]. The modified hyaluronan forms a gel-like substance, which is then extruded through a sieve, forcing the gel into smaller particles. The smallest particles are packaged as low-density Hylaform Fine Line, the medium-sized particles are labeled as Hylaform, and the large particles form the high-density Hylaform Plus (approved by the FDA in October 2004). These products last from 3 to 4 months and all contain HA concentrations of 5.5 mg/mL. Hylaform Fine Line, not yet approved by the FDA, is indicated for fine wrinkles and injection in the superficial dermis. Hylaform is best suited to the body of the lips and the smoker's lines, whereas Hylaform Plus is more appropriate for deeper lines and improving cheekbone and cheek volume. Hylaform and Hylaform Plus are the only animal-derived sources of HA that are FDA approved in the United States. The longer chains of HA may make them less "sticky" (imagine long, cooked strands of spaghetti as compared with short ones), so they tend to diffuse more than the bacterially derived fillers. This factor accounts for the ease of injection and softness of the product. For this reason, Hylaform is the author's filler of choice in the body of the lips, although the longevity of this product may be shorter than that of other, bacterially derived HA fillers.

Bruising, sterile abscesses, and short-lived erythema are among the rare side effects. Patients who are allergic to products of avian origin should not use these products. Other contraindications for the Hylaform products are similar to those for bovine-derived fillers, including allergic background, autoimmune and inflammatory disorders, history of anaphylactic reactions, immunosuppressant therapy, pregnancy, and breastfeeding [9]. The randomized, double-blind multicenter clinical trials of Hylaform and Hylaform Plus that resulted in approval of both products by the FDA also demonstrated that they are comparable in efficacy and safety to Zyplast.

Captique

Captique (Allergan Corporation, Irvine, California) is an HA that is produced by Genzyme Corporation in the same manner as Hylaform. The only difference between these products is the source: the HA in Captique is of bacterial origin, so the strands of HA are shorter. Consequently, Captique is slightly stiffer than Hylaform and is more difficult to inject with a 30-gauge needle. Using a 27-gauge needle will make this product much easier to inject. Its longevity is purported to be from 4 to 6 months.

Restylane

Restylane (Q-Med, Uppsala, Sweden; Medicis, Scottsdale, Arizona) is a bacterially derived HA product used successfully in Europe since the early 1990s and approved in more than 60 countries. In December 2003, the FDA approved Restylane for the treatment of nasolabial folds. Approval followed the results of a randomized, double-blind multicenter comparison of Restylane and Zyplast that demonstrated the HA product to be equivalent to Zyplast [44]. Specifically, the trial showed that both products were equally safe in the treatment of nasolabial folds, producing similar short-lived side effects, such as erythema, swelling, and bruising [45]. Although Restylane is of bacterial origin, it is easy to inject, because unmodified (uncross-linked) HA has been added to the syringe to increase the ease of extrusion. Restylane is slightly stiffer than the other HA products, which makes it useful in areas such as deep wrinkles. Perlane, not yet approved by the FDA, is identical to Restylane except that the gel particles are larger, imparting greater longevity. Duration trials on Restylane and Perlane have not been performed, but anecdotally physicians report lasting results for 6 to 9 months with Restylane and longer with Perlane. Swelling and bruising are common. Slowly injecting the HA may reduce the risk of inducing inflammation; systemic prednisone can also mitigate swelling in patients [46,47].

Juvéderm

Juvéderm (Allergan Corporation, Irvine, California) is composed of HA obtained from bacterial fermentation through a process similar to Restylane. Heat and filtration eliminate the bacteria. HA strands are cross-linked using the same cross-linking agent that is used to produce Restylane and Perlane (BDDE).

Juvéderm is said to differ from Hylaform and Restylane insofar as it is a homogeneous gel, not one broken into smaller particles. Reduced surface area is exposed with the homogeneous gel as compared with the nonhomogeneous products, which is believed to decrease hyaluronidase activity and result in a longer-lasting correction [48]. In addition, the homogeneity of the gel is believed to render it more biocompatible, because it creates less friction with dermal tissues on injection, provoking less inflammation. Comparative clinical trials have not yet been conducted to consider the relative inflammation associations across the three HA product lines. As seen with Restylane, unmodified HA is added to the Juvéderm syringe to increase the ease of injection.

The five Juvéderm products (Juvéderm 18, Juvéderm 24, Juvéderm 24 HV, Juvéderm 30, and Juvéderm 30HV) vary by the amount of HA per milliliter, the amount of cross-linking in the product, and the regularity of its cross-linking. The FDA recently approved Juvéderm 24 HV, Juvéderm 30, and Juvéderm 30HV.

Of note, the use of any HA product results in more swelling and bruising than do procedures using collagen products. This observation is ascribed to the structural similarity of HA and heparin, suggesting that HA products may cause an anticoagulant effect, leading to more bruising [49,50]. Pretreating patients with a collagen-containing agent, because of the platelet-aggregating effect produced by collagen, may result in reduced bruising [39]. In the author's practice, we first treat large areas of the patient's face with Sculptra (Dermik Laboratories, Berwyn, PA) diluted with 5 mL of sterile water and 1 mL of lidocaine (Xylocaine) 1% with epinephrine. (Technique and placement are beyond the scope of this article.) After the Sculptra treatments have been performed and massaged as directed, the collagen and HA products may be added. It is believed, though not yet proved, that the epinephrine will decrease the degree of bruising seen with the HA fillers.

Although the HA filling agents represent exciting options in the expanding armamentarium of soft tissue augmentation, they are not likely to replace collagen products in these procedures. Collagen products will continue to play an important role in these cosmetic procedures, probably because of the strong correlation between high type I collagen levels and younger-looking skin. In addition, CosmoPlast demonstrates greater capacity to provide structural support to treated areas, particularly the vermilion border of the lips, than do HA products. However, CosmoPlast cannot provide the same volume as the HA products, which potently bind water. For this reason, combining these different forms of filling agent can be useful. Using HA fillers in combination should result in less swelling and bruising than is observed with HA fillers alone, because of the effects of lidocaine [40].

Injection techniques

Over the last several decades, techniques for the use of collagen fillers have been honed through sheer and expansive repetition. Injection techniques have evolved as these products have become increasingly and exceedingly popular. Injection techniques vary to some extent from practitioner to practitioner, but certain guidelines must always be followed. Although some physicians continue to use just one type of dermal filler, innovation in products and techniques has resulted in the current approach of layering different dermal and subcutaneous fillers.

As in other procedures, it is important to make the patient as comfortable as possible. This principle facilitates the augmentation injection for the physician as well as the patient. In most circumstances, it is ideal to have the patient sitting upright, which renders the treatment area more accessible for marking or delineating, as well as for treating. If the patient is reclining, most of the dermal defects will be minimized, potentially leading to undercorrection and patient dissatisfaction. Limiting pain is also a key aspect of the procedure. Most patients are able to tolerate injection of these agents without regional anesthesia because of the presence of lidocaine in most collagen-containing dermal filling agents. In addition, pretreatment of the patient with lidocaine containing Sculptra can have the bonus of providing anesthesia. Topical anesthetics may also be used. When using fillers in combination, one injects the Sculptra first and vigorously massages it with an agent such as Arnica (Boiron, Lyon, France) to prevent bruising. Collagen is then placed and gently massaged. HA is placed last and should be minimally massaged to minimize bruising and swelling. In the author's experience with hundreds of patients, this technique is very effective and results in little to no down-time.

After the treatment area has been visually delineated, the depth of the defect must be ascertained so that the most suitable filling agent may be selected. CosmoDerm or Zyderm is the most suitable agent for treating very superficial epidermal defects. A serial puncture technique is used to inject these fillers into the papillary dermis, where a temporary, minor blanching of the skin is noted at the injection site, revealing accurate placement of the product. It is important to be vigilant about overcorrection with Zyderm, which causes localized swelling, although it typically subsides in approximately 24 hours. Overcorrection with CosmoDerm is less likely, because swelling with this product is less common than it is with Zyderm. Massage is usually not necessary when using these agents. If approved by the FDA, Restylane Fine Line, Hylaform Fine Line, and Juvéderm 18 may be substituted to treat these areas. CosmoDerm and Zyderm are also options for the correction of superficial perioral rhytides. The vermilion border of the lips is better treated with CosmoPlast or Restylane because of its thicker consistency. Adding botulinum toxin to the perioral area can enhance and prolong the results of the other fillers.

Placed into the middle or deeper layers of the dermis, CosmoPlast and Zyplast are indicated for slightly deeper defects and furrows. Injection of either material should be performed with a 30-gauge needle at a 45° angle with the skin, medial to the wrinkle. The filler may be injected using either the serial puncture technique or the linear threading technique. CosmoPlast is effective for lip enhancement when placed in the vermilion border with one of the HA products in the body of the lip (Figs. 1–4). The nose is also a suitable site for CosmoPlast injection; it may be used for the ridges in the columella or for lifting of the nasal tip (Figs. 5 and 6). The presence of lidocaine in CosmoPlast, which imparts anesthesia, renders the HA injection more tolerable in combination procedures. Overcorrection is unnecessary with either CosmoPlast or Zyplast.

Combining specific products

CosmoPlast and CosmoDerm for the lips

These two collagen products may be combined for effective lip augmentation. Minimal swelling and bruising result from this procedure, as compared with the use of HA products. This result may be due to the inclusion in these collagen products of lidocaine, which can inhibit the activation of eosinophils that may contribute to swelling and bruising

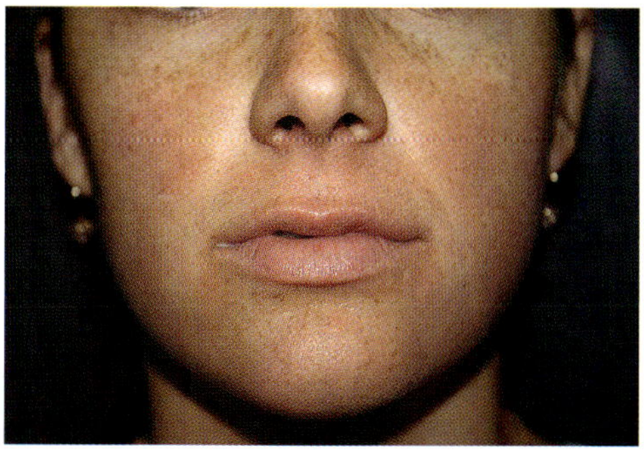

Fig. 1. Lips prior to correction. Note notching in left upper lip that makes upper lip asymmetric.

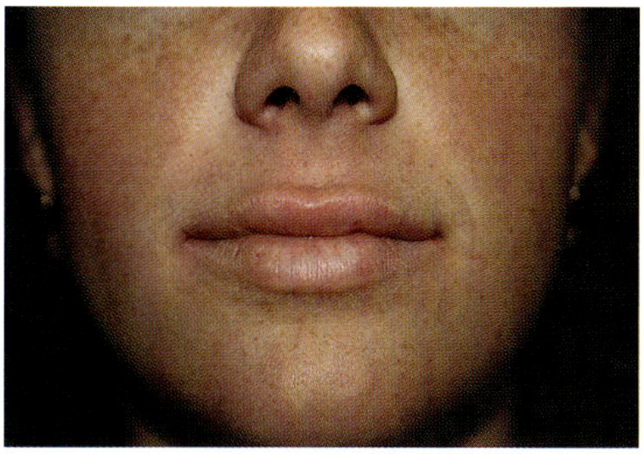

Fig. 2. After application of CosmoPlast to the vermilion border only. Note that swelling of lip body occurs, although implant was placed only in the vermilion border.

[40]. To achieve this correction, CosmoPlast should be injected into the vermilion border and CosmoDerm injected into the body of the lips.

CosmoPlast and CosmoDerm for facial lines

CosmoPlast should be injected just medial to the wrinkle at the middermis level. A 45° angle is ideal to achieve the proper placement in the dermis. If superficial lines remain after the placement of CosmoPlast, CosmoDerm may be injected in the upper dermis to erase the remaining wrinkles. Because swelling is minimal with these products, it is important neither to over- nor to undercorrect with them.

CosmoPlast and Hylaform, Juvéderm, or Restylane for the lips

Although it is not approved for this use, CosmoPlast is the ideal filler for the vermilion border of the lips. The structure that is necessary to impart an aesthetically desirable altitude to the lip lining is provided by the collagen in CosmoPlast. An HA product may then be used to thread the body of

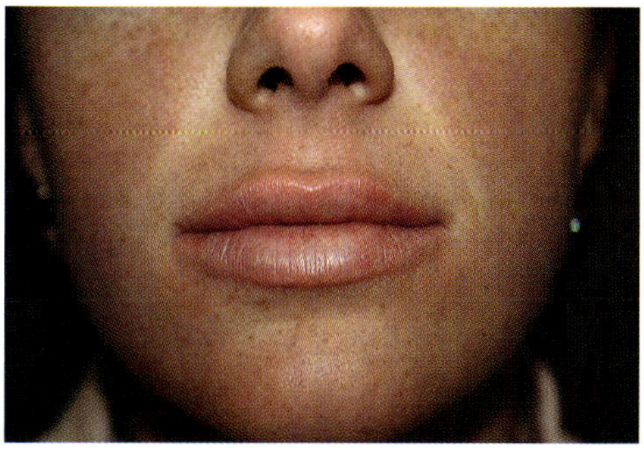

Fig. 3. After application of Hylaform in the body of the upper and lower lips.

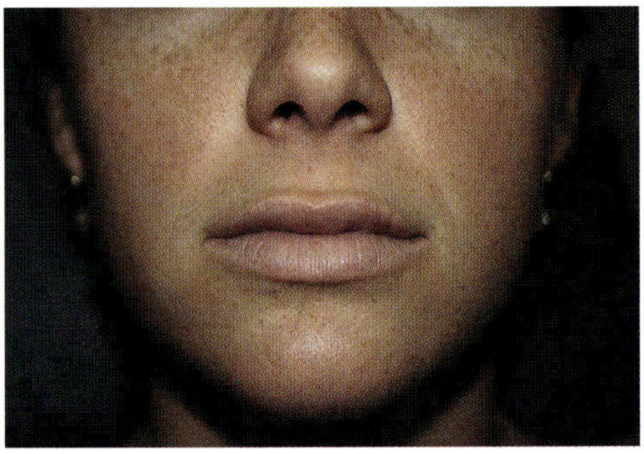

Fig. 4. Twenty-four hours later. Swelling has ceased. It is now apparent that the notching in the left upper lip is improved.

the lips, because the HA draws water into the lips, imparting the volume that is lost with aging.

CosmoPlast and Hylaform, Juvéderm, or Restylane for facial lines

Combining CosmoPlast with an HA filler may be ideal for treating facial lines. CosmoPlast should be injected into the middermis until a correction of about 75% is achieved. With the treatment area numbed by the lidocaine in the collagen product, Hylaform, Juvéderm, or Restylane may then be injected in the same plane as the CosmoPlast. In this combination therapy, collagen confers the needed structure, and HA provides the desired volume. All facial lines other than glabellar furrows may be treated with this technique. Because of the risk for necrosis, glabellar lines should be treated with fillers that are less dense, such as CosmoDerm II. Botox (Allergan, Inc., Irvine, CA) is probably best in this instance. If residual lines remain in the

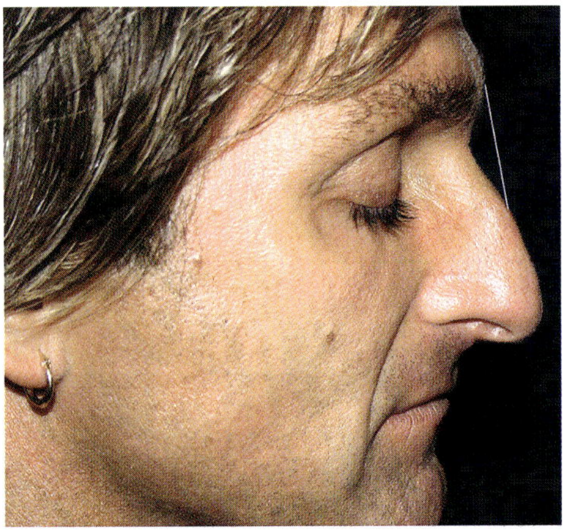

Fig. 5. Nose prior to injection of collagen in the upper nasal bridge and just above the central philtrum.

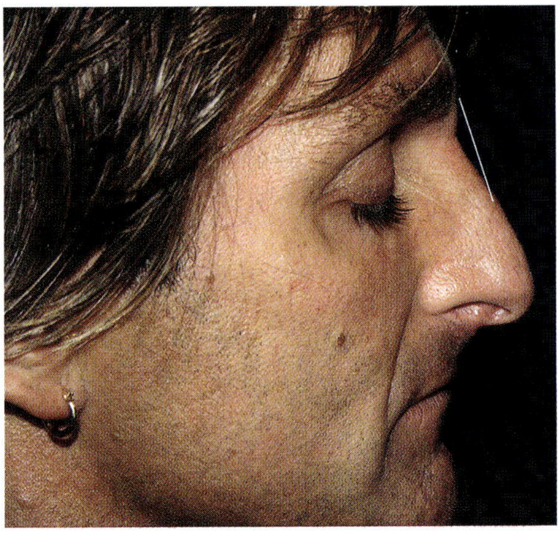

Fig. 6. After injection of CosmoPlast. Note that the angle of the nasal bridge has decreased and that the nasal tip is higher.

glabellar area after treatment with Botox, CosmoDerm I or II or Zyderm may be injected in this area to complete the correction.

Hylaform, Juvéderm, or Restylane and CosmoDerm for facial lines

Another effective means of achieving an optimal correction may be to use an HA product first to treat facial lines, injecting into the middermis with a technique similar to that used with CosmoPlast and Zyplast, and then layering over with CosmoDerm when superficial lines remain. Currently, CosmoDerm and Zyderm I are the only fillers available in the United States that are intended for injection into the superficial dermis to treat superficial lines, but Hylaform Fine Line and Restylane Fine Line will most likely be available in the near future.

Sculptra, Cosmoplast, and Hylaform, Juvéderm, or Restylane

Sculptra, known as New Fill in Asia and Europe, is approved for the treatment of HIV-induced lipoatrophy but can be used off label for the treatment of wrinkles. It is not a true dermal filler but rather a dermal stimulator that encourages the fibroblasts to make collagen. Sculptra may be injected into the jowls, cheekbone area, temples, nasolabial folds, and perioral and periorbital lines. It is recommended that one be well trained in this procedure before attempting it, because the learning curve is steep. Once injected, Sculptra is massaged for several minutes. CosmoPlast or Zyplast or both may then be injected into the vermilion border, the bridge of the nose, and the columella, used to raise the corners of the mouth, and injected into deep wrinkles. The collagen product is then gently massaged. The massage is crucial in the corner of the mouth and the vermilion border to avoid clumping. Finally, an HA product of choice may be used in the body of the lips (choose a soft one), as well as in the cheekbones, nasolabial folds, and any other needed areas.

Summary

Collagen, HA, and elastin are all lost in the aging process. Replacement of these components improves the appearance of the skin. At this time, no elastin-containing fillers are on the market. Collagen- and HA-containing fillers may be used together to produce a superior aesthetic result. The techniques and products used vary from physician to physician, because this is an art as well as a science. It is important to remember to combine these treatments with a good skin care routine, including sunscreen, antioxidants, and retinoids, to slow the aging process [51].

References

[1] Epstein EH Jr. (Alpha1(3))3 human skin collagen. Release by pepsin digestion and preponderance in fetal life. J Biol Chem 1974;249(10):3225–31.

[2] Fenske NA, Lober CW. Structural and functional changes of normal aging skin. J Am Acad Dermatol 1986;15(4 Pt 1):571–85.

[3] Lavker RM. Structural alterations in exposed and unexposed aged skin. J Invest Dermatol 1979; 73(1):59–66.

[4] Lovell CR, Smolenski KA, Duance VC, et al. Type I and III collagen content and fibre distribution in normal human skin during ageing. Br J Dermatol 1987;117(4):419–28.

[5] Fisher GJ, Datta SC, Talwar HS, et al. Molecular basis of sun-induced premature skin ageing and retinoid antagonism. Nature 1996;379(6563): 335–9.

[6] Fisher GJ, Wang ZQ, Datta SC, et al. Pathophysiology of premature skin aging induced by ultraviolet light. N Engl J Med 1997;337(20):1419–28.

[7] Griffiths CE, Russman AN, Majmudar G, et al. Restoration of collagen formation in photodamaged human skin by tretinoin (retinoic acid). N Engl J Med 1993;329(8):530–5.

[8] Talwar HS, Griffiths CE, Fisher GJ, et al. Reduced type I and type III procollagens in photodamaged adult human skin. J Invest Dermatol 1995;105(2):285–90.

[9] Bergeret-Galley C. Comparison of resorbable soft tissue fillers. Aesthetic Surgery Journal 2004;24: 33–46.

[10] Piacquadio D, Larson NE, Denlinger JL, et al. Hylan B gel (Hylaform) as a soft tissue augmentation material. In: Klein AW, editor. Tissue augmentation in clinical practice: procedures and techniques. New York: Marcel Dekker; 1997.

[11] Haake A, Holbrook K. The structure and development of skin. In: Freedberg IM, Eisen AZ, Wolff K, et al, editors. Fitzpatrick's dermatology in general medicine. Vol. 1 5th edition. New York: McGraw Hill; 1999. p. 89–90.

[12] Ghersetich I, Lotti T, Campanile G, et al. Hyaluronic acid in cutaneous intrinsic aging. Int J Dermatol 1994;33:119–22.

[13] Milewicz DM, Urban Z, Boyd C. Genetic disorders of the elastic fiber system. Matrix Biol 2000;19(6):471–80.

[14] Escoffier C, de Rigal J, Rochefort A, et al. Age-related mechanical properties of human skin: an in vivo study. J Invest Dermatol 1989;93: 353–7.

[15] Boente MC, Winik BC, Asial RA. Wrinkly skin syndrome: ultrastructural alterations of the elastic fibers. Pediatr Dermatol 1999;16:113–7.

[16] Neuber F. Fettransplantation. Chir Kongr Verhandl Dsch Gesellch Chir 1893;22:66.

[17] Klein AW, Elson ML. The history of substances for soft tissue augmentation. Dermatol Surg 2000;26(12):1096–105.

[18] Baumann L. Soft tissue augmentation. In: Baumann L, editor. Cosmetic dermatology: principles and practice. New York: McGraw-Hill; 2002. p. 155–72.

[19] Clark DP, Hanke CW, Swanson NA. Dermal implants: safety of products injected for soft tissue augmentation. J Am Acad Dermatol 1989; 21(5 Pt 1):992–8.

[20] Klein AW. Injectable collagen. In: Moschells SL, Hurley HJ, editors. Dermatology. Philadelphia: WB Saunders; 1992. p. 2455–61.

[21] Hanke CW, Coleman WP III. Dermal filler substances. In: Asken S, Alt TH, Hanke CW, et al, editors. Cosmetic surgery of the skin. St. Louis (MO): Mosby-Year Book; 1997. p. 217–30.

[22] Hanke CW, Higley HR, Jolivette DM, et al. Abscess formation and local necrosis after treatment with Zyderm or Zyplast collagen implant. J Am Acad Dermatol 1991;25(2 Pt 1):319–26.

[23] Stegman SJ, Chu S, Armstrong RC. Adverse reactions to bovine collagen implant: clinical and histologic features. J Dermatol Surg Oncol 1988;14:39–48.

[24] Elson ML. The role of skin testing in the use of collagen injectable materials. J Dermatol Surg Oncol 1989;15(3):301–3.

[25] Castrow FF 2nd, Krull EA. Injectable collagen implant—update. J Am Acad Dermatol 1983; 9(6):889–93.

[26] Siegle RJ, McCoy JP Jr, Schade W, et al. Intradermal implantation of bovine collagen. Humoral immune responses associated with clinical reactions. Arch Dermatol 1984;120(2):183–7.

[27] Klein AW, Rish DC. Injectable collagen update. J Dermatol Surg Oncol 1984;10(7):519–22.

[28] Klein AW. In favor of double testing. J Dermatol Surg Oncol 1989;15(3):263.
[29] Baumann LS, Kerdel F. The treatment of bovine collagen allergy with cyclosporin. Dermatol Surg 1999;25(3):247–9.
[30] Moody BR, Sengelmann RD. Topical tacrolimus in the treatment of bovine collagen hypersensitivity. Dermatol Surg 2001;27(9):789–91.
[31] Cukier J, Beauchamp RA, Spindler JS, et al. Association between bovine collagen dermal implants and a dermatomyositis or a polymyositis-like syndrome. Ann Intern Med 1993;118(12):920–8.
[32] Hanke CW, Thomas JA, Lee WT, et al. Risk assessment of polymyositis/dermatomyositis after treatment with injectable bovine collagen implants. J Am Acad Dermatol 1996;34(3):450–4.
[33] Rosenberg MJ, Reichlin M. Is there an association between injectable collagen and polymyositis/dermatomyositis? Arthritis Rheum 1994; 37(5):747–53.
[34] Elson ML. Injectable collagen and autoimmune disease. J Dermatol Surg Oncol 1993;19(2): 165–8 [discussion: 170].
[35] Lemperle G, Gauthier-Hazan N, Lemperle M. PMMA-microspheres (Artecoll) for long-lasting correction of wrinkles: refinements and statistical results. Aesthetic Plast Surg 1998;22(5): 356–65.
[36] Cohen SR, Holmes RE. Artecoll: a long-lasting injectable wrinkle filler material: report of a controlled, randomized, multicenter clinical trial of 251 subjects. Plast Reconstr Surg 2004;114(4): 964–76 [discussion: 977–9].
[37] Broder KW, Cohen SR. ArteFill: a permanent skin filler. Expert Rev Med Devices 2006;3(3):281–9.
[38] Lemperle G, Romano JJ, Busso M. Soft tissue augmentation with Artecoll: 10-year history, indications, techniques, and complications. Dermatol Surg 2003;29(6):573–87 [discussion: 587].
[39] Perret S, Eble JA, Siljander PR, et al. Prolyl hydroxylation of collagen type I is required for efficient binding to integrin alpha 1 beta 1 and platelet glycoprotein VI but not to alpha 2 beta 1. J Biol Chem 2003;278(32):29873–9.
[40] Okada S, Hagan JB, Kato M, et al. Lidocaine and its analogues inhibit IL-5–mediated survival and activation of human eosinophils. J Immunol 1998;160(8):4010–7.
[41] Baumann L. CosmoDerm/CosmoPlast (human bioengineered collagen) for the aging face. Facial Plast Surg 2004;20(2):125–8.
[42] Larsen NE, Pollack CT, Reiner K, et al. Hylan Gel biomaterial: dermal and immunologic compatibility. J Biomed Mater Res 1993;27:1129–34.
[43] Balazs EA, Bland PA, Denlinger JL, et al. Matrix engineering. Blood Coagul Fibrinolysis 1991; 2(1):173–8 [review].
[44] Transcript from the General and Plastic Surgery Devices Panel of the Medical Devices Advisory Committee of the FDA on November 21, 2003. Available at: http://www.fda.gov/ohrms/dockets/ac/03/transcripts/4004T1.htm and http://www.fda.gov/ohrms/dockets/ac/03/transcripts/4004T1_01.htm.
[45] Narins RS, Brandt F, Leyden J, et al. A randomized, double-blind multicenter comparison of the efficacy and tolerability of Restylane versus Zyplast for the correction of nasolabial folds. Dermatol Surg 2003;29:588–95.
[46] Malson T, Lindqvist B. Ge of crosslinked hyaluronic acid for use as a vitreous humor substitute. European Patent 0185070; 1985.
[47] Narins RS. Soft tissue augmentation course. American Academy of Dermatology, February 2004.
[48] Vercruysse KP, Marecak DM, Marecek JF, et al. Synthesis and in vitro degradation of new polyvalent hydrazide cross-linked hydrogels of hyaluronic acid. Bioconjug Chem 1997;8:686–94.
[49] Barbucci R, Lamponi S, Magnani A, et al. The influence of molecular weight on the biological activity of heparin like sulphated hyaluronic acids. Biomaterials 1998;19(7–9):801–6.
[50] Pandolfi M, Hedner U. The effect of sodium hyaluronate and sodium chondroitin sulfate on the coagulation system in vitro. Ophthalmology 1984;91(7):864–6.
[51] Baumann L. How to prevent photoaging. J Invest Dermatol 2005;125(4):xii–iii.

ELSEVIER
SAUNDERS

CLINICS IN PLASTIC SURGERY

Clin Plastic Surg 33 (2006) 597–601

Legal Ramifications of Off-Label Filler Use

David J. Goldberg, MD, JD[a,b,c,*]

Cosmetic surgeons use a variety of devices and drugs in an off-label manner. Botox (Allergan, Irvine, CA) and Restylane (Medicis, Scottsdale, AZ) are Food and Drug Administration (FDA) cleared for glabelar use and nasolabial folds, respectively; thus, treatment for any other anatomic location is defined as "off-label use." Fillers, in contrast to botulinum toxin injections, are considered by the FDA to be devices rather than drugs. In this manner fillers are much like lasers and light-based devices. Many lasers have been FDA cleared for one purpose and yet are used by physicians for a variety of purposes. This is also considered off-label use. Botulinum toxins, like a whole variety of medications, may also be FDA cleared for one purpose, yet can be used in an off-label manner. Although the FDA approval process for drugs and devices can be quite different, the principles that apply to off-label use apply to both drugs and devices.

There are a variety of FDA-cleared dermal fillers currently in use in the United States. Restylane, Hyalform (Inamed, Santa Barbara, CA), and Captique (Inamed) are hyaluronic acid dermal fillers currently FDA cleared for nasolabial folds. As described in the preceding paragraph, use of these fillers for the lip or crow's feet is considered off-label use (Figs. 1 and 2). Similarly, Sculptra (Dermik, Belwyn, PA) is a poly L lactic acid that is FDA cleared for use in HIV lipoatrophy. However, this agent is more commonly used for off-label, non–FDA-cleared, facial volume enhancement in non-HIV patients. Finally, Radiesse (Bioform, Franksville, WI) is a calcium hydroxyapatite material that has more than one noncosmetic FDA clearance, yet this filler is most commonly used for cosmetic purposes, an off-label use (Figs. 3 and 4). Use of Juvederm, expected to be FDA approved in the near future, cannot at the time of this writing be used in an off-label manner.

The regulation of off-label drugs and devices is a complicated and controversial area of the law. Regulators must protect patients' safety without interfering with physicians' practice of medicine or manufacturers' First Amendment rights. This article will first explore manufacturer promotion of off-label use of both drugs and devices. Then both the legality of dermatologist off-label use as well as the medical legal issues of off-label use of fillers will be discussed.

Before one explores the legalities of off-label use of dermal fillers, it is important to distinguish between those fillers that are used in an off-label manner and those that have no FDA labeling at all. The latter group of fillers has not received FDA clearance for any purpose. Examples of such fillers at the time of this writing are Juvederm, Artefill, and Aquamid. Although very popular in many countries, such fillers cannot be used in the United States for any purpose in any legal manner. If and when these fillers are FDA cleared, their use will be legal. However, until such FDA approval happens, the use of such fillers is illegal. Importing such fillers from outside the United States may be associated with both civil and criminal liability. Further, if an

[a] Skin Laser and Surgery Specialists of NY/NJ, 115 East 57th Street, Suite 710, New York, NY 10022, USA
[b] Department of Dermatology, Mount Sinai School of Medicine, 5 East 98th Street, New York, NY 10029, USA
[c] Fordham Law School, 140 West 62nd Street, New York, NY 10023, USA
* Skin Laser and Surgery Specialists of NY/NJ, 115 East 57th Street, Suite 710, New York, NY 10022.
E-mail address: drdavidgoldberg@skinandlasers.com

doi:10.1016/j.cps.2006.08.003
plasticsurgery.theclinics.com

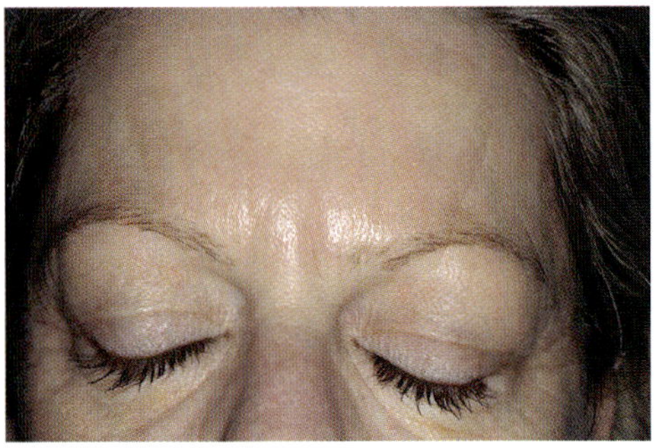

Fig. 1. Glabelar area before injection of Captique, a legal, off-label use of this filler.

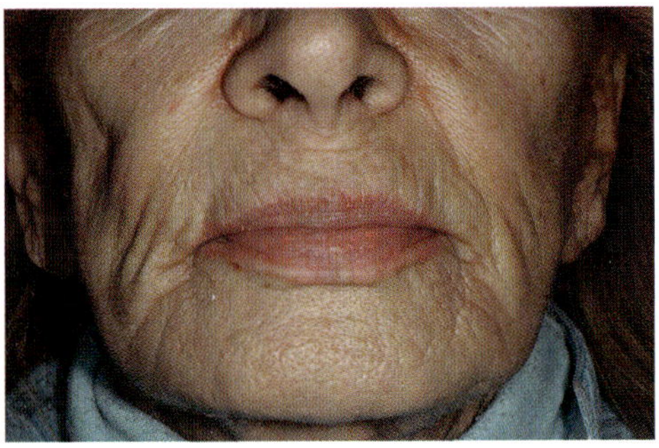

Fig. 3. Lips before injection of Cosmoderm, a legal, off-label use of this filler.

untoward event occurs following the use of such a filler, it is unlikely that such a problem will be covered by medical malpractice policies (Fig. 5).

Off-label drug and device use refers to the very common practice of using a drug, or a device, in a manner or for a reason not currently approved by the FDA [1]. An off-label drug or device is not necessarily dangerous. In fact, for many diseases, off-label use of many medications is the best or even the only course of treatment available. Pharmaceutical and device manufacturers, however, with certain minor exceptions, are not permitted to encourage off-label use of their products. Although this area of the law has developed considerably over the past decade, several important issues remain unsettled. Are restrictions on off-label promotion good policy? Does government regulation promote patient safety or simply interfere with the legitimate practice of medicine?

As described above, an "off-label drug" is simply a medication and an "off-label filler" is simply a filler (a device) used for a condition or in a manner not appearing on the FDA-approved label [2]. Indeed, almost every consumer is familiar with off-label medicines. The American Medical Association reported in 1995 that approximately half of all prescriptions were written for off-label uses [3]. Moreover, the General Accounting Office (GAO) has testified that 90% of cancer drug use, 80% of pediatric use, and 80% to 90% of drugs used to treat rare diseases are prescribed off-label [4]. Perhaps the best-known example is aspirin. For years, physicians prescribed aspirin to reduce the risk of heart attacks [5]. However, the FDA did not approve such usage until 1998. A less celebrated example is Fen-Phen [6]. Both fenfluramine ("Fen") and phentermine ("Phen") were approved by the FDA for weight loss [7]. However, many physicians ignored fenfluramine's labeling by having some patients use the medicine for more than a year when it was only labeled for a duration of a "few weeks," and by combining the two drugs even though neither label discussed using the drugs in tandem. Many patients suffered heart valve damage as a result [8]. Most recently [9], OxyContin, a powerful medication approved for moderate to severe chronic pain, generated considerable controversy when it was prescribed for all types of discomfort [10]. Off-label use, therefore, comes in a variety of forms. While some instances are widely accepted, and doctors could be accused of malpractice if they did not prescribe the use [11,12], others are dangerous and are not an appropriate part of medical care. This same principle would be applied to dermal fillers. In a discussion of fillers used as cosmetic volume-enhancing agents, in non-HIV+

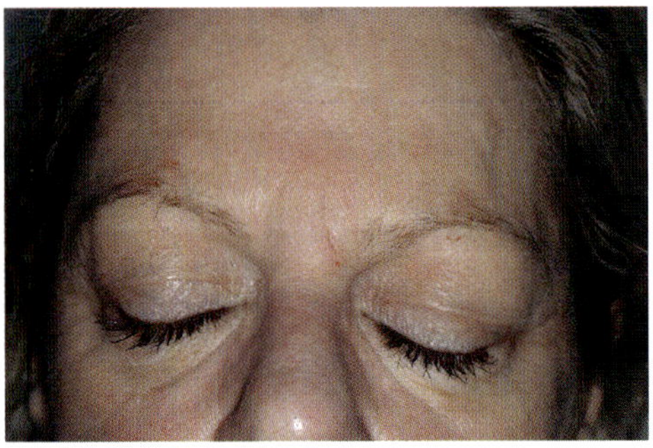

Fig. 2. Glabelar area after injection of Captique.

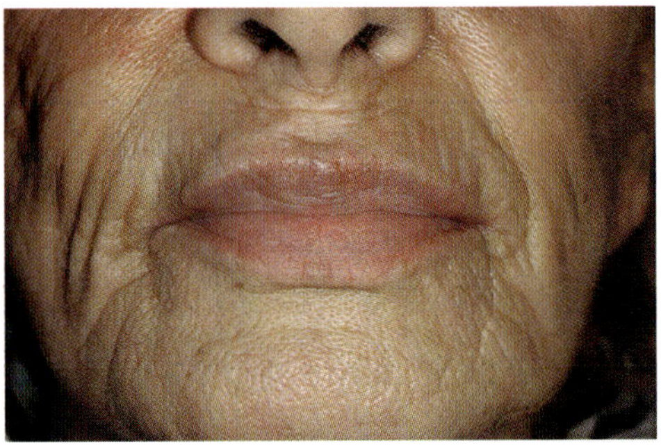

Fig. 4. Lips after injection of Cosmoderm.

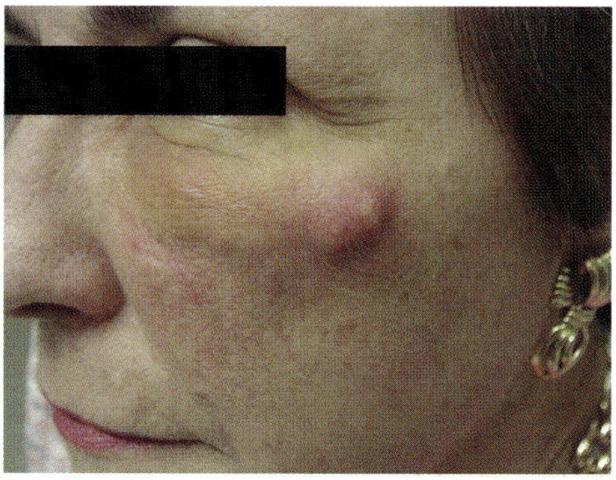

Fig. 5. Complication after Aquamid, a filler without FDA clearance. Use is illegal and will not be covered by medical malpractice insurance.

patients it might be considered malpractice if poly-L- lactic acid and calcium hydroxyapatite were not part of the discussion. This is true even though both of these agents are being used in an off-label manner for these purposes.

Three kinds of off-label uses have been described: off-label use in its truest form, off-label marketing, and off-label prescription. Off-label use occurs when a consumer uses a drug in a manner inconsistent with its label. Frequently, this entails a patient changing the dosage amount or frequency, combining the drug with others, using the medicine to treat an unapproved condition, or giving the medicine to someone for whom it was not prescribed. It is nearly impossible to monitor off-label use and Congress has never attempted to outlaw its practice. It is also an off-label use that does not apply to dermal fillers.

Off-label marketing is, in fact, regulated by the FDA. The FDA has clearly ruled that manufacturers cannot market their products for purposes, to users, in dosages, or in combinations other than FDA-approved ones. While recent legislation has created certain exceptions to this blanket prohibition [13], the promotion of drugs or devices for off-label uses remains both highly regulated and controversial.

In 1938 Congress passed the Food, Drug, and Cosmetics Act (FDCA). In doing so, the members of the 75th Congress firmly established the federal government's role in regulating the pharmaceutical industry and ensuring the safety of the nation's prescription drug supply. Congress made it clear that while it intended to regulate production and distribution of prescription drugs, it did not wish to regulate the practice of medicine. As courts have noted, new uses for both drugs and devices are often discovered after the FDA approves the package inserts that explain a drug's approved uses. Congress would have created havoc in the practice of medicine had it required physicians to follow the expensive and time-consuming procedure of obtaining FDA approval before putting drugs to new uses. Thus, Congress exempted the practice of medicine from the FDCA so as not to limit a physician's ability to treat patients.

However, this distinction—between the practice of medicine on one hand and the promotion of drugs or devices on the other—has been a difficult one to maintain. As mentioned above, federal regulations prohibit pharmaceutical manufacturers from encouraging off-label use of their products, but if physicians learn of and then use off-label uses, no law has been violated [13]. The problem is that the medical device/ prescription drug industry and physicians work hand in hand to deal with everyday medical problems.

Amending the FDCA in 1962, Congress placed the regulation of devices under the jurisdiction of the FDA. Bovine collagen, with its FDA clearance in the 1980s, represented the first time the FDA dealt with today's dermal filler. Its FDA clearance was for nasolabial folds. All approved fillers, after bovine collagen, have sought similar labeling and therefore its use on other anatomic areas represents an off-label use.

As part of a broad overhaul of the FDA [13], Congress passed the Food and Drug Administration Modernization Act of 1997 (FDAMA) [13]. While not removing all restrictions on off-label marketing, the law does facilitate the distribution of information from the pharmaceutical industry to physicians. The FDAMA, which has been described as the most important change in drug regulation in 20 years, seeks to balance the interests of physicians, and correspondingly of their patients, to obtain legitimate information about drug uses against FDA's continued interest in ensuring that manufacturers continue to study drug effectiveness.

Significantly, the FDAMA does permit manufacturers of an FDA-approved drug or device (such as a dermal filler) to distribute information about new uses for that drug. However, there are restrictions. Manufacturers can distribute an unchanged reprint of a peer-reviewed journal article or a reprint of a reference publication that experts in the field consider scientifically sound. The peer-reviewed articles must be indexed in the *Index Medicus*. The distribution must be accompanied by (1) a disclosure statement that identifies the reprint as information regarding an unapproved use, (2) notes that the manufacturer has sponsored the distribution, and (3) identifies any author or consultant who has financial ties to the manufacturer. Finally, manufacturers may only distribute information from journals that have a publicly stated policy of disclosing authors' conflicts of interest.

Under the new law, manufacturers can only distribute the information to health care practitioners, pharmacy benefit managers, health insurance issuers, group health plans, and government agencies. Of note, manufacturers may not distribute these reprints to patients and consumer groups.

The final category of off-label prescription, in contrast, occurs when a doctor prescribes a drug or uses a device in a manner inconsistent with its FDA-approved label. For example, a physician may prescribe a drug for a disease other than the ones listed on the label, in an unapproved dosage, for unapproved duration, or in an unapproved combination with other medicines. The doctor may also prescribe the drug to groups, such as children or pregnant women, for whom the FDA has not approved the drug's usage. While it would be easier to enforce a ban on off-label prescription than it would be for off-label use, Congress has long deferred to a physician's superior medical judgment to prescribe medicine or use devices. This is also the category of off-label "use" that applies to the everyday use of dermal fillers by dermatologists for purposes other than those on the original labeling. Numerous decisions support this approach, which emphasizes physician autonomy and discretion within an otherwise rigorous regulatory environment [14].

It should be noted that there is no question as to the legality of off-label use for dermal fillers [14]. The only dispute concerns the appropriateness of filler manufacturers promoting the off-label aspects of their product. All would agree that off-label use is widespread in the medical community and often is essential to giving patients optimal medical care. Medical ethicists, the FDA, and most courts have recognized this fact [15]. Off-label use often represents "state-of-the-art" treatment, and the FDA asserts that "good medical practice and patient interests require that physicians use commercially available drugs, devices, and biologics, according to their best knowledge and judgment." Thus, the term "off-label" is merely a regulatory description of a drug; it is a legal status not a medical fact.

Furthermore, it is important not to interpret the phrase "unapproved use" to mean "disapproved use" [16]. The FDA does not take a position on the safety of an off-label use; rather, the agency leaves that determination to the individual doctor as part of his or her practice of medicine. This position has been stated repeatedly. For example, in a 1972 pronouncement, the FDA declared that once a drug or device has left a manufacturer's warehouse a physician may, as part of the practice of medicine, lawfully prescribe a different dosage of a drug for his patient, or may otherwise vary the conditions of use of the drug or device from those approved in the actual manufacturer-provided labeling [17]. Ten years later, the FDA again stressed that off-label use is accepted medical practice, and FDA-approved labeling should be used for informational purposes only. Physicians have embraced this freedom, and off-label use has become an accepted method of treatment in medical practice [17].

However, when a medical malpractice lawsuit evolves over the off-label use of a filler, the situation can become murky. This is best explained by the following hypothetical situation:

Dr Cosmetic is a regular user of calcium hydroxyapatite filler injections for cheek volume enhancement in non-HIV+ individuals. His consent form very clearly stipulates that nodule formation can occur after the placement of this filler. Dr Cosmetic has never seen this problem before and knows that it is rare. Unfortunately, such nodule formation occurs in one of his patients, a television actress. Although the nodules are more palpable than visible, they clearly do distort the shape of the patient's cheeks. She sues Dr Cosmetic. The basis of the lawsuit is that Dr Cosmetic used the calcium hydroxyapatite in an off-label manner.

Dr Cosmetic will look for an expert witness to testify that his method of treatment was consistent with what is commonly done by other cosmetic surgeons. Evidence of the standard of care in a specific malpractice case includes laws, regulations, and guidelines for practice. These represent a consensus among professionals often with a focus on the medical literature including peer-reviewed articles and lectures at national meetings [18]. Dr Cosmetic is likely to find such an expert and will probably not lose his case.

In summary, off-label use of dermal fillers is commonly performed in the United States. When "off-label" is defined as use of a currently FDA-approved dermal filler in an off-label manner, consistent with that done by other physicians, there is no basis for liability. Such use of dermal fillers is perfectly legal.

References

[1] Furrow BF, Greaney TL, Johnson SH, et al. Liability in health care law. 3rd edition. St Paul, MN: West Publishing Co.; 1997.

[2] Beck JM, Elizabeth D. FDA, off-label use, and informed consent: debunking myths and misconceptions. Food Drug Law J 1998;71:58–70.

[3] Veronica H. Off-label prescribing: legal implications. J Leg Med 1999;20:365–78.

[4] Final Report on the Activities of the House Committee on Government and Oversight, 104th Cong, 2d Sess, 104 H Rep 874 (Section 2) (January 2, 1997):114.

[5] Oliphant J. FDA's new drug war industry fights for alternative uses of approved products. Legal Times. January 10, 2000:1.
[6] Elliot v A.H. Robins Co. (*In re* NY County Diet Drug Litig), 691 NYS2d 501 (App Div 1999).
[7] Rheingold PD, Rheingold DB. Offense or defense? Managing the off-label use claim. Trial March 2001;52.
[8] O'Reilly J, Dalal A. Off-label or out of bounds? Prescriber and marketer liability for unapproved uses of FDA-approved drugs. Ann Health L 2003; 12:295–300.
[9] Salbu SR. Off-label use, prescription, and marketing of FDA-approved drugs: an assessment of legislative and regulatory policy. Fla Law Rev 2002;51:18–21.
[10] Ford MA. Another use of oxycontin: the case for enhancing liability for off-label drug marketing. BU Law Rev 2003;83:429–61.
[11] Noah L. Informed consent and the elusive dichotomy between standard and experimental therapy. Am J Law Med 2002;28:361–99.
[12] Rhone-Poulenc Rorer Pharms Inc v Marion Merrell Dow Inc, 93 F3d 511, 514 n3 (8th Cir 1996).
[13] Food and Drug Administration Modernization Act of 1997, Pub L No 105–115, 111 Stat 2296.
[14] US General Accounting Office. Off-label drugs: reimbursement policies constrain physicians in their choice of cancer therapies. Washington, DC: US General Accounting Office; 1991. Publication GAO/PEMD-91–14, 11.
[15] Buckman Co v Plaintiffs' Legal Comm, 531 US 341–351, 2001.
[16] Proctor v Davis, 682 NE2d 1203, 1213 (Ill App), 1997.
[17] Food and Drug Administration. Use of approved drugs for unlabeled indications. FDA Drug Bulletin, April 1982.
[18] Hyams AL, Shapiro DW, Brennan TA. Medical practice guidelines in malpractice litigation: an early retrospective. J Health Polit Policy Law 1996;21:289–307.

ELSEVIER
SAUNDERS

CLINICS IN
PLASTIC
SURGERY

Clin Plastic Surg 33 (2006) 603–606

Index

Note: Page numbers of article titles are in **boldface** type.

A

B

C

D

doi:10.1016/S0094-1298(06)00095-2
plasticsurgery.theclinics.com

E

F

G

H

S

T

V

W

Z